More Advance Praise for

THE HEALTHY BRAIN

"Aileen Burford Mason's common-sense book is sweetly written—engaging, lively and persuasive. As a medical/ nutrition work, it is helpful and practical. Anyone who toils away at any job really should read the chapter 'Into the Workplace,' which is not only instructive; it is an absolute tonic."

JOHN DOYLE,

author of *The World Is a Ball: The Joy, Madness and Meaning of Soccer*

"The human brain has a big appetite—but is yours going hungry? Anchored in the latest science and full of fascinating case histories, this easy-to-use guide to boosting your brain power explains the crucial link between what we eat and our memory, mood, cognition and ability to handle stress. It makes total sense!"

MARNI JACKSON,

author of *Pain: The Science and Culture of Why We Hurt*

THE
HEALTHY
BRAIN

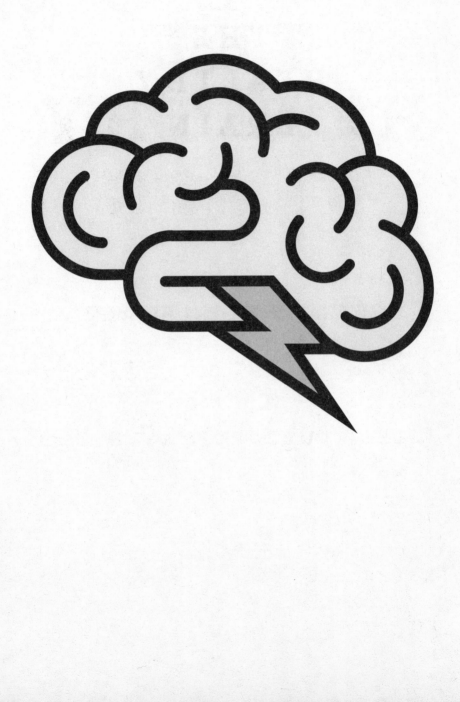

THE HEALTHY BRAIN

OPTIMIZE BRAIN POWER AT ANY AGE

AILEEN BURFORD-MASON, PhD

PATRICK CREAN EDITIONS
HarperCollins*Publishers*Ltd

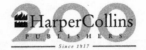

The Healthy Brain
Copyright © 2017 by Aileen Burford-Mason.
All rights reserved.

Published by Patrick Crean Editions,
an imprint of HarperCollins Publishers Ltd

First Canadian edition

HarperCollins books may be purchased for educational, business,
or sales promotional use through our Special Markets Department.

HarperCollins Publishers Ltd
2 Bloor Street East, 20th Floor
Toronto, Ontario, Canada
M4W 1A8

www.harpercollins.ca

Library and Archives Canada Cataloguing in Publication
information is available upon request.

ISBN 978-1-44344-778-2

Printed and bound in the United States of America
LSC/C 10 9 8 7 6 5 4 3 2 1

In memory of my friend and mentor,
Dr. Ursula Martius Franklin
(1921–2016)

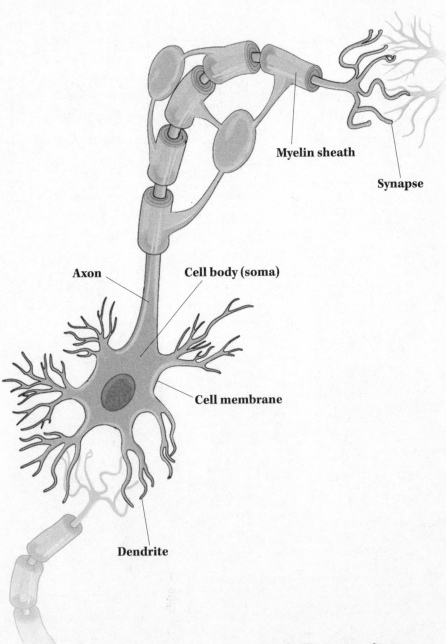

Myelin sheath

Synapse

Axon

Cell body (soma)

Cell membrane

Dendrite

Figure. Illustration of a neuron

We are drowning in information, while starving for wisdom.
The world henceforth will be run by synthesizers, people able to
put together the right information at the right time, think critically
about it, and make important choices wisely.

E.O. WILSON, PhD,
Consilience: The Unity of Knowledge

Contents

Introduction...1

PART 1: The Brain—A User's Guide

Chapter 1: A Journey across Time.............................9
Chapter 2: Nature versus Nurture............................25
Chapter 3: The Nutrition-Cognition Connection...............41
Chapter 4: Vitamins, Minerals and Brain Function 55

PART 2: When the Brain Stalls

Chapter 5: Alzheimer's and Dementia: Our Greatest Fears..........77
Chapter 6: This Is Your Brain on Stress.....................95
Chapter 7: Brain Injuries: Trauma and Stroke 111

PART 3: Back to the Beginning

Chapter 8: Brain under Construction: Diet and Pregnancy..........129
Chapter 9: Supplements and Pregnancy.......................141
Chapter 10: Prenatal Planning: A Checklist..................157

PART 4: Making Brains Last a Lifetime

Chapter 11: The Learning Brain: Diet and Academic Success.........169
Chapter 12: Into the Workplace..............................181
Chapter 13: What to Do If Memory Fails 197

PART 5: Planning Strategies

Chapter 14: Shopping Smarts: Budget-Conscious Choices
            at the Grocery Store............................213
Chapter 15: Supplement Protocols............................227

Appendix: Fruit and Vegetable Diary 247

Acknowledgements...251
Endnotes...253
Index..277

Introduction

If the human brain were so simple that we could understand it,
we would be so simple that we couldn't.

EMERSON M. PUGH, in G.E. PUGH,
THE BIOLOGICAL ORIGIN OF HUMAN VALUES

These days it's hard to open a newspaper or magazine without reading an article about the fragile state of our collective mental health. Autism is on the rise; teenagers are taking their own lives. Debilitating depression and anxiety are commonplace. Baby boomers face the frightening possibility of dementia not too far down the road. In Canada, one in five people will develop a mental health illness during their lifetime.

Other stories lament the deterioration of our food, and how inadequate diets are contributing to the huge burden of chronic disease our strained health-care budgets are coping with. But only the rare media story makes the link between deteriorating mental health and the food we eat. As the most metabolically active organ of the body, the brain has nutritional needs that are ten times higher than those of any other organ. So it may be the first organ to falter when nutrients are undersupplied. Some failures in brain chemistry are temporary and reversible. For example, we lose focus and concentration when we go too long without food and our blood sugar drops. This is an easy fix: just eat. But what the brain cannot withstand is the continuous underprovision of the nutrition it needs—the indispensable factors in food that keep it functioning.

According to the World Health Organization, dementia now affects 47.5 million people worldwide, and these numbers will skyrocket as populations age.[1] In Canada, figures from the Alzheimer's Society show

1

that more than half a million people are living with the disease, with twenty-five thousand new cases being diagnosed every year.[2] However, scientists now admit that dementia is not an inevitable part of the aging process. It's a lifestyle disease, for which poor nutrition and lack of exercise are the major risk factors. Pharmaceutical approaches to treatment so far have been spectacular failures, which means our best option is taking steps to prevent the onset of dementia.

Current efforts to prevent dementia are aimed at those on the cusp of acquiring it—the middle-aged—who are urged to stop smoking, reduce alcohol intake, exercise daily and improve their diet. However, if we want our brains to last a lifetime, we need to start a lot earlier. In fact, as you will see in this book, much of our brain power is laid down in utero—the nine months before we are born. Like other diseases of aging, dementia may be a late-stage presentation of undernutrition at earlier life stages, with pregnancy a period of particular vulnerability.

While we can do nothing about the nourishment we received before we were born, with careful diet and appropriate supplements, any brain can be coaxed into improved performance. Regardless of our early nutritional history, there are many ways to enhance brain power at later stages of life. We *can* overcome the genetic impact of our nutritional heritage. Conversely, even the smartest brain will suffer when the nutrients it needs to function are regularly underconsumed. No matter how smart a brain we were born with, it will not last a lifetime without careful feeding.

Moreover, considering evidence that stress and intense intellectual or physical work also dramatically increase the need for many nutrients, we are all likely to suffer from dietary shortfalls from time to time. Many of us are pushing our brains to work hard while at the same time denying them the sustenance they need for efficient functioning. Think of the student, the ambitious executive, the athlete or the weekend warrior. Any of these individuals might be underperforming because they are short of protein, vitamin C or magnesium. As you'll see from this book, both hard-working bodies and active brains can benefit from the use of nutritional supplements.

Just as a highway underpass that is not regularly inspected for maintenance and repair may begin to collapse, discharging dangerous chunks of concrete onto cars below, so we cannot assume that the brain will work well without proper maintenance and continuous attention to its food needs. It is the cumulative effect over many years of incorrect feeding that leads to the final collapse of the brain.[3]

In the twenty-first century, medicine faces a dilemma. Although poor nutrition is driving waves of obesity, diabetes and heart disease, there is little emphasis on nutrition in medical training. On average, doctors in North American medical schools receive 19.6 hours of nutritional education.[4] Blink and you miss it. Consequently, many doctors graduate with no more nutritional knowledge than a high school student. In the meantime, the whole field of nutritional research is exploding. The research literature is now so vast and complex that it has become an almost herculean task to fill the knowledge gap between those who keep abreast of developments in the field and those who do not.

But while their doctors are ignoring the role of nutrition in health, patients have been doing their homework, educating themselves on the Internet. Many are better informed on the latest research than their physicians. Often they find out by themselves that unexplained symptoms they've been experiencing can be solved by fine-tuning their diets and adding nutritional supplements. Not surprisingly, such patients are frustrated when the role of nutrition is ignored in their treatment— when research that is relevant to their care is either not known by their physicians or dismissed as irrelevant.

The professional training of dieticians is another problem, since it is currently rooted in the concept that there's no need to take extra vitamins as supplements. If we eat well, so the story goes, we will be healthy; if we follow official healthy eating guidelines, we will get all the essential nutrients we need. However, government statistics in Canada and the United States show widespread deficiencies of many key nutrients, even in those who consider themselves to be healthy eaters.[5] In Canada, a Senate committee found that Canada's Food Guide needs a drastic makeover and does not provide sound nutritional guidance: "Canada's Food Guide has been at best ineffective and at worst enabling with respect to the rising levels of unhealthy weights and diet-related chronic diseases in Canada."[6]

Since the earliest days of vitamin research, it has been clear that we differ from one another in the amount of each nutrient we need, often dramatically. To quote from the *Heinz Handbook of Nutrition*, published in 1959, "In the light of contemporary genetic and physiologic knowledge the typical individual is more likely to be one who has average needs with respect to many essential nutrients but who also exhibits some nutritional requirements for a few essential nutrients which are far from average."[7]

Is the idea that we each have our own unique needs for vitamins an outmoded concept? Is it okay to continue believing that the current officially sanctioned recommendations for vitamins (recommended daily allowances) fit all our needs? No. On the contrary, new sciences are emerging that show that, if anything, we have underestimated just how individual we are when it comes to nutritional requirements. A long roster of new scientific disciplines—nutrigenomics, metabolomics and many other "-omics"—is confirming what we have known for decades: there is no one-size-fits-all.

Understanding these new disciplines requires a deep understanding of biochemistry, genetics and nutrition in all their complexity. According to one recent review, "It is often difficult, even for educated professionals, to appreciate their relevance to the practice of preventive approaches for optimising health, delaying onset of disease and diminishing its severity."[8] How much more difficult is it for those not educated in nutrition and oblivious of rapidly evolving research?

Nutritional guidelines in all developed countries have avoided grappling with this uncomfortable truth. Instead, recommendations are based on a single intake of nutrients for everyone, with minor adjustments for men and women and for different age groups. But far from satisfying the nutritional needs for most of us, current recommended intakes fail to deliver optimal intakes for any of us.

While this book is neither a textbook about the brain nor a primer on nutrition, it does attempt to show how they interact. Ultimately, all parts of the brain are intimately connected and work in harmony to control moods, focus and attention. All participate in memory formation, storage and retrieval. Similarly, all essential nutrients need to be present in the body at all times, in optimal amounts and properly balanced. There are no magic nutritional bullets.

While this may sound complicated, this book gives step-by-step guidance on how to implement dietary changes and select appropriate supplements. The immediate payoff of adopting these strategies is a noticeable increase in brain vitality—better mood, focus, creativity and workplace performance, and an improved capacity to enjoy life, sleep soundly and cope well under stress. And in the long term, the dietary changes I outline are those that have shown the most promise in helping us dodge Alzheimer's disease or other forms of dementia.

One last comment. Readers familiar with current trends in brain research will be aware of the immense interest in what we now call the "microbiome"—the many trillions of microbes living within us and on us. In the first few days of life, we are colonized by a huge collection of microorganisms—bacteria, viruses and fungi. Although the human gut microbiome is relatively stable over time within each individual, alterations occur when we are exposed to prolonged stress or drugs like antibiotics or those used in chemotherapy. The microbiome can also change rapidly in response to poor diet, gastrointestinal illness and travel.[9]

Alterations in the composition and diversity of these microbes have been shown to influence our vulnerability to heart disease, autoimmune diseases, weight gain, metabolic syndrome and type 2 diabetes. By interacting with the central nervous system, the gut microbiome also impacts how our brains function. We know that a healthy microbiome plays an integral role in an infant's normal neurological development. Adult brain health is also influenced: research is beginning to establish links between this largely hidden microbial world and levels of anxiety and depression, and even conditions like autism, bipolar disorder and schizophrenia.

What is not exactly clear at this point is how we can manipulate these complex microbial communities: a lot more research needs to be done before we know for sure how to harness them for improved mental and physical health. For this reason, I feel it premature to include a discussion of the microbiome in this book. But stay tuned. This complex field is moving fast.

PART 1

The Brain—A User's Guide

CHAPTER 1

A Journey across Time

I, George Bush, President of the United States of America, do hereby proclaim the decade beginning January 1, 1990, as the Decade of the Brain. I call upon all public officials and the people of the United States to observe that decade with appropriate programs, ceremonies, and activities.

It is July 17, 1990. In the White House, George H.W. Bush has just signed Presidential Proclamation 6158, designating the decade beginning January 1, 1990, as the Decade of the Brain. The previous fifteen years have seen extraordinary advances in brain imaging technology; it is now possible to look inside a living brain and visualize how it works. With innovative technology in place, the time is ripe for a grand political gesture—an initiative that will see an unprecedented flow of government and private funds into brain research.

This new initiative has tremendous appeal. Doctors are hopeful that the injection of substantial funds into brain research will generate a better understanding of what goes wrong in a range of mental health disorders—from depression and autism to schizophrenia, epilepsy, drug addiction and dementia—and lead to new and improved methods for treatment and prevention. And since mental illness consumes a substantial and growing chunk of health care spending, governments and health economists definitely agree.

For the rest of us, this decade begins an enduring love affair with brain science. Compared to all previous history, knowledge about the brain and its inner workings doubles during the Decade of the Brain. New findings are enthusiastically and often sensationally covered by the media. Scientists respond to increased media attention by writing popular books explaining their highly technical work—books that in turn create a better-informed lay audience eager to learn more.

Our curiosity is piqued. How does the brain control our actions, our thoughts, our feelings? Can all this new science make us smarter, or alter the course of lifelong depression or anxiety? Can we begin to understand what was going on in the brain of a beloved friend or family member who took their own life? Can the growing body of information on the brain and its workings finally help us figure out what makes us "us"?

Command central

The quest to understand the human brain and how it controls our physical and emotional functioning is as old as written human history. The ancient Greeks had little understanding of basic brain physiology and anatomy, and the arguments of the day were mainly philosophical: What part of the brain housed "common sense"? Which areas controlled memory, reason and imagination? What was the relationship between the brain and the soul, spirit or mind? Where was the soul located?

Hippocrates (c. 460–c. 375 BC) believed the brain was the seat of intelligence and responsible for all our senses. "Men ought to know that from the brain and from the brain only arise our pleasures, joys, laughter and jests, as well as our sorrows, pains, grieves and tears," he declared. However, not many years later the views of another prominent and influential Greek, Aristotle (384–22 BC), would dominate. According to Aristotle and his followers, it was not the brain but the heart that defined the essence of who we were. The heart alone was the source of our intelligence. The brain was merely a cooling device, useful only because it acted as a safety valve to release the copious amounts of heat generated by our hard-working hearts.

Not needed on the journey

The ancient Egyptians also placed little value on the brain. In common with many early civilizations, the Egyptians practised mummification and preserved the body after death. They believed that the physical body would be resurrected in the afterlife, and so it had to be conserved intact, and as perfectly as possible.

The process of mummification was long and laborious. The internal organs were removed first because they quickly decomposed. These were separately embalmed. The only organ left intact inside the body was the heart. As the source of the intellect and emotion it would be vitally important in the afterlife. The body, together with its undisturbed heart, was then dehydrated and embalmed. The other internal organs were later returned to their original locations and the body wrapped in many layers of linen strips. Amulets were placed between the layers to protect the body during its journey into the next world.

The only organ discarded in the process was the brain. The ancient Egyptians believed they could get along perfectly well in the afterlife without a brain.

Moving away from superstition

The Islamic Golden Age (in the seventh to thirteenth centuries) saw the emergence of many new ideas in technology and medicine, and fanciful assumptions gradually began to give way to a more systematic and scientific approach to unravelling the brain and its secrets. The great Arab physicist and pioneering scientific thinker Alhazen (965–1040), best known for his descriptions of how the eye transmits images to the brain, was the first to suggest that any ideas about how the brain works should be discarded unless they could be confirmed by observation and experiment. "The seeker after truth is not one who studies the writings of the ancients and puts his trust in them, but rather the one who suspects his faith in them, and questions what he gathers from them; the one who submits to argument and demonstration and not the sayings of human beings whose nature is fraught with all kinds of imperfection and deficiency," he wrote.

This was the beginning of what we know today as the scientific method.

During the Renaissance, many scientists were also accomplished artists. As meticulous dissections began to reveal human anatomy in greater detail, each new discovery needed to be documented and illustrated. And so the arts and sciences flourished side by side. The most famous example of this marriage of art and science is artist and inventor Leonardo da Vinci (1452–1519). A self-taught anatomist, da Vinci initially studied physiology and anatomy so he could reproduce the structure of the human body more faithfully in his paintings. But he also had an interest in the structure of the brain, and made detailed and beautiful drawings of it.

At this time, labels were given to different parts of the brain that we still use today. The cerebrum (Latin for "brain"), located in the front area of the skull, occupies about two-thirds of the brain's total mass. Consisting of two hemispheres, a left and a right, the cerebrum controls higher brain functions like thought and action. The cerebellum (Latin for "little brain") is located at the back of the skull and controls movement and balance. The medulla lies in front of the cerebellum and regulates the involuntary processes of the body, including blood pressure, heart rate, digestion and breathing.

When wrinkles are a good thing

One of the earliest and best-known anatomy textbooks, *De humani corporis fabrica* (On the workings of the human body), published by Andreas Vesalius in 1543, was the first book to clearly distinguish two different types of brain tissue, based on colour: the grey matter or cerebral cortex, which forms the outer layer of the brain, and the central white matter.

This text also includes the first accurate drawings of the surface of the brain: the many wrinkles that form grooves (sulci) and ridges (gyri) on its outer aspect. The early anatomists had thought these convolutions were random, and similar to the worm-like coils of intestine that spilled out of the abdomen when they cut it open. Vesalius himself did not think these peaks and troughs were anything special: "There is nothing unusual about man's brain, and these convolutions appearing in its substance are also to be found in the brain of the ass, horse, ox and other animals which I have examined."

By the end of the sixteenth century, however, it was clear that in this regard, Vesalius was mistaken. The surface convolutions are neither random nor in loose coils, but are firmly attached to the deeper parts of the brain. And they *are* more extensive among the higher animals.

Comparing the brains of different species, as the cerebrum gets larger, the convolutions become increasingly more elaborate. Engravings from the period show a clear evolutionary progression: the beaver brain is smooth, the fox brain has five convolutions, the horse brain has more indentations than the sheep, and the elephant brain more than the horse. But no animal brain shows more complex convolutions than the human brain.

Bumps, lumps and personality

In the early part of the nineteenth century Franz Joseph Gall (1758–1828), a German anatomist, was a name on everyone's lips. Skilled in anatomy and dissection, he was the first to identify the cranial nerves—twelve pairs of nerves that exit the brain through openings in the skull, rather than through the spinal column. Some of these nerves, he showed, control sensory organs, some control muscles, and others are connected to glands or internal organs like the heart and lungs. This discovery was an important and lasting contribution made by Gall to the evolving science of neurology.

But Gall's work on the cranial nerves was not what attracted the most attention—rather, his theory of phrenology made him famous and wildly popular with the general public. The brain, in Gall's theory, was not one organ but many, each found at a specific site in the brain's convolutions, and each controlling different emotions and mental functions. Because the shape of the skull followed the convolutions of the brain itself, he believed, the size and shape of the skull—its bumps, lumps and indentations—could be used to identify individual personality traits and mental strengths and weaknesses.

Gall examined the heads of groups of people he felt occupied the behavioural extremes of society—criminals and clergymen, for example—and mapped out the regions he thought governed particular qualities like deviousness and criminality, honesty and conscientiousness, and even artistic gifts like musicality. Feeling each other's bumps, or having one's bumps read, became a popular pastime—a Sunday afternoon parlour game. Even Queen Victoria is reported to have invited a phrenologist to read the heads of her many children, looking for insight into their talents and temperaments.

By the mid-nineteenth century phrenology was big business, especially in America, where phrenology institutes were established in most major cities. Phrenologists claimed they could diagnose illness and calculate future disease risk. Couples used it to test their compatibility before marriage, and businesses to screen job applicants. It was even suggested that politicians be tested by a phrenologist before standing for public office. Expressions we still use today, such as "highbrow," "lowbrow" and "you need your head examined," come from that period.

The demise of phrenology and the birth of psychology

The only trouble was that Gall, for all his skills in dissection, was not a good scientist. His original work had been highly selective, reporting only the subjects that confirmed his theories and dismissing all evidence to the contrary. French physiologist Marie-Jean-Pierre Flourens (1794–1867) made it known that he was angered by what he considered to be the deception of the public by pseudoscience. He was eventually commissioned by Napoleon Bonaparte to test Gall's popular theories. Using animal experiments, Flourens proved Gall wrong, and phrenology was dismissed as so much hocus-pocus.

However, these public disagreements about phrenology and the relationship between the shape of the skull and brain function eventually led scientists back to thinking about the nature of the many wrinkly convolutions on the cerebral cortex. Why were they more numerous and complex in humans compared to other mammals? What were the evolutionary pressures that led to their formation? Carl Wernicke (1848–1905) suggested that they were the result of increasing brain size. As we got smarter and our brains increased in size, brain growth was limited by the size of our skulls. When the brain could not expand outwards because of space restrictions, it expanded inwards.

By the end of the nineteenth century, detailed maps showing the structure and function of the various parts of the brain began to emerge.

The forebrain, containing the cerebral cortex, was the seat of feelings, learning and memory. Information from our eyes, ears and other sensory organs was processed first by the midbrain and then relayed to the forebrain. Language was shown to be localized in the left hemisphere of the brain, while involuntary functions like breathing and digestion were located in the hindbrain, with most of the cranial nerves.

In the late 1800s, renewed interest in how the mind affected behaviour gave birth to a new discipline—psychology. German physiologist Wilhelm Wundt (1832–1920) was one of the first to take a systematic approach to studying abnormal mental states, using measurable phenomena like attention span and reaction time. Mental processes, he argued, could be analyzed and tabulated in much the same way a chemist analyzes and categorizes chemical compounds.

Wundt also made an important contribution to evolving scientific methodology. He insisted that all experiments should be carried out in carefully controlled conditions and thoroughly described so that they could later be reproduced by other scientists. If a result wasn't reproducible, it was unlikely to be true.

Interestingly, recent scientific analyses suggest that as much as 50 per cent of scientific endeavours published today—even in leading medical journals—may be unreproducible and therefore potentially misleading.[1]

An accidental experiment

In the Warren Anatomical Museum on the campus of Harvard University Medical School, a glass case houses an odd group of items: the skull of a man, an iron mask of the man's face and a long metal rod. The skull and face mask belonged to Phineas Gage, a construction worker. The metal rod is a tamping iron, used to cram dynamite into crevices and holes bored into rocks before detonating it to level the rock face for building purposes.

In 1842, twenty-five-year-old Gage is the foreman of a crew cutting a new railroad bed through the undulating granite of Vermont. While he is using the metal rod to pack dynamite into the rock, the dynamite suddenly explodes, sending the rod skywards. The rod pierces Gage's cheek, penetrating his brain through the frontal lobe, blasts its way through his skull and finally exits, coming to rest upright in the earth some feet away.

Amazingly, Phineas Gage lives. Immediately after the accident he can walk and talk, and he takes himself back to his hotel, where a doctor later digs pieces of his shattered skull out of his brain and dresses his wound. Initially he survives a coma, a brain infection and periods of delirium, all interspersed with periods of lucidity. However, his convalescence over the next four years is slow and erratic. It is to the credit of his attending physician, Dr. John Martin Harlow, that Gage survives at all: few doctors of the day would have been skilled enough to drain a brain abscess successfully.

Physically Phineas Gage recovers well, although blind in one eye and with one side of his face paralyzed. But by all accounts he is temperamentally a changed man. Where once he was responsible and a quiet and industrious worker, Gage is now surly and combative. Fired by his employers, he finds it difficult to hold down any job. This famous case, now found in countless neuroscience textbooks, was an important milestone in the study of the brain's anatomy and its links to behaviour. Not only did it show that personality is linked to the frontal lobe, but it illustrated how personality can change if that area of the brain is damaged.

Recently, researchers at UCLA re-examined the case of Phineas Gage using imaging data of his skull. The tamping iron, they found, would have caused widespread damage to the white matter connections throughout Gage's brain. Because we now know that white matter connects various regions of the brain that must work together for reason and memory, the researchers speculate that the destruction of this white matter disrupted the connectivity between the various brain regions. This damage caused the behavioural changes poor Phineas experienced.[2]

Phineas Gage died in San Francisco after an epileptic seizure aged thirty-seven, twelve years after the accident.

The microscope reveals more secrets

Meanwhile, the evolving science of microscopy was revealing yet more secrets of the brain. In the mid-1700s, English scientist Robert Hooke (1635–1703) had been using a magnifying glass to examine a thin sliver of cork. What he saw suggested that cork was composed of numerous tiny enclosed chambers, closely packed together. Since they were similar in shape to the small rooms or cells inhabited by monks in monasteries, he named these structures cells.[3] Hooke had just discovered the basic building block for all life forms, from plants to animals and humans.

As optical science evolved, the magnifying glass gave way to the microscope. Although crude at first, the microscope revealed the anatomy of the brain in greater and more intimate detail than ever before. New methods were invented to "fix" the delicate, jelly-like brain tissue by soaking it in alcohol or formaldehyde so that it didn't disintegrate when handled and could be cut into thin, almost transparent slices. A variety of staining techniques were developed to add colour and highlight different internal structures within the cells.

But science rarely progresses in straightforward, join-the-dots steps. More often than not conflicting views give rise to warring factions, each asserting that its interpretation of scientific observations is correct. The nascent science of neuroanatomy was no different. Although scientists agreed that the cell was the basic unit of all living things, the cell theory was not believed to apply to the brain and nervous system. Spanish pathologist Santiago Ramón y Cajal (1852–1934) first suggested that cells seen in the brain called neurons were the basic functional units of the brain and nervous system, and a growing number of other scientists thought so too. But another group thought that it was not these cells but the dense network (reticulum) of fine fibres seen under the microscope that controlled the brain's workings.

Pass it on

We now know that these fibres were projections of the neurons and not independent of them. Each neuron has three distinct regions. The largest and most obvious central part is the cell body, or soma, which houses the nucleus. Projecting outwards from this are many spindly branches called dendrites, which themselves branch, often multiple times, and are collectively known as the dendritic tree. Dendrites pick up chemical signals from other neurons and transport them to the cell body, which then relays them on to other cells. It is the job of a distinctly different protrusion from the cell body, the axon or nerve fibre, to make sure that the message is passed on.

Each neuron has many dendrites but only one axon, some of which are very long—a nerve fibre carrying messages from the spinal column to a muscle in the toe, for example, may be up to a metre in length. The grey matter of the brain contains most of the cell bodies and dendrites as well as some axons, whereas the white matter is composed largely of the information-handling axons, with fewer cell bodies. The fact that the cell body, the dendrites and the axon are all part of one cell was not clear during most of the nineteenth century because each of the parts had been observed and studied separately.

Since the mature brain looks so incredibly complex under the microscope, Cajal thought it might be easier to examine earlier stages of life when the brain was not so well developed. A new and improved silver-based stain had recently been developed, and he used this to stain sections of the brains of chicken embryos and show that the cell body, its dendrites and axon were all part of the same cell—the neuron. Cajal had a lot in common with Leonardo da Vinci: as well as being a fine anatomist, he was an accomplished artist. His beautifully detailed pen and ink drawings can be seen at the Cajal Institute in Madrid.

Santiago Ramón y Cajal shared the 1906 Nobel Prize for Medicine with Italian pathologist Camillo Golgi, who had invented the silver stain that Cajal used.

Brain waves

While it was all very well to try to understand brain anatomy by looking at specimens through the microscope, these static images revealed nothing about brain activity. Then, in the late nineteenth century, spontaneous electrical signals were observed emanating from the brain. These could be recorded by placing electrodes directly onto the exposed brains of rabbits and dogs. Because the signals fluctuated in intensity, they were called brain waves.

German physiologist and psychiatrist Hans Berger (1873–1941) invented the first machine to record brain waves in humans, the electroencephalograph (EEG). There was no need to expose the brain, he found. Electrodes could be attached directly to the scalp. The changes in voltage EEGs recorded were very small—ten thousand times smaller than that of a single AA battery—but now at last the activity in the brain could be monitored. We could begin to see this complex and mysterious organ at work.

The EEG marked a momentous development in neurology and is still as useful today as when it was first invented. Animal experiments showed that there was a spike in brain waves just before an epileptic seizure, so during World War Two EEGs were used to screen pilots for epilepsy and their fitness to fly planes. In the 1950s, the EEG showed for the first time that brain waves during sleep are very similar to the brain waves of subjects who are awake. Up to this point the brain was thought to be idle during sleep, which was considered simply a period of down-time for a tired brain. But the EEG told a different story. During sleep our brains were as busy as during any period of wakefulness.

In later chapters we will explore sleep in more detail, since we now know a good night's sleep is critical for a host of metabolic and cognitive functions, including learning and memory. And we will see that a good night's sleep depends on how well our brains are fed.

The war of the "sparks and soups"

One important question remained unanswered: How do neurons communicate? By the middle of the twentieth century everyone agreed that neurons were physically separated from one another and were not fused into continuous networks as the reticulists of the nineteenth century had believed. A gap called the synapse exists between the tail end of the axon and the dendrite of another neuron. The main question was how signals make their way across this gap. How was information transmitted from one neuron to another? Was the signal electrical or chemical in nature?

Pharmacologists believed that nerves communicate by releasing a chemical at the synapse, while neurophysiologists believed that an electrical "spark" jumps from one neuron to another, transmitting information. As it turned out, both camps were right. Transmission between nerves indeed occurs by way of direct movement of molecules from one neuron to another. Two scientists, Otto Loewi and Henry Dale, received the 1936 Nobel Prize for demonstrating that chemical messages (neurotransmitters) are emptied into the synapse from the terminal end of the axon and that these messenger molecules enable rapid communication between neurons, and from the brain to organs and muscles.

However, the pharmacologists had hardly finished their victory dance when electrical synapses were discovered. First identified in the 1950s in the primitive brain of the crayfish, they were later found to be present in all nervous systems. Although electrical synapses are a distinct minority, they have essential features that distinguish them from their chemical cousins. First, they are built for speed, and transmission is extraordinarily fast—a fraction of a millisecond. Electrical synapses are necessary for lightning-quick responses such as reflex actions. Second, electrical synapses control synchronicity, where groups of neurons fire simultaneously to magnify a response. It is electrical synapses that orchestrate the burst of hormones, such as adrenaline or cortisol, that pour into our circulatory systems when we are stressed.

Both electrical communication and chemical communication between neurons is essential. They are complementary, working side by side for normal physiological functioning.

The other brain cells

While most attention had focused on neurons as the primary players in the brain, another type of cell had also been observed. At first they were not even recognized as distinct cells at all, because they looked like an oily slick filling the gaps between neurons. Later, using special fixatives and stains, it was shown that they were independent cells. Considered of little functional importance and assumed simply to provide physical support for neurons, holding them in place, they were named glial cells. (*Glia* is Greek for "glue.")

However, early neuroscientists underestimated the role glial cells play. Some types of glial cells—the oligodendrocytes—send out projections that wrap themselves around axons, forming a layer of insulation called the myelin sheath. This insulation allows faster transmission of electrical signals from one neuron to another and serves as a protective covering for the axon. The white matter of the brain largely consists of myelinated axons that connect different parts of the grey matter together. Myelin is what gives white matter its characteristic colour.

The oligodendrocytes are responsible for maintaining the axon in good working order, feeding it, removing debris, and repairing and replacing myelin. If the myelin is lost, the axon becomes damaged. Scars form, reducing the efficiency with which the axon connects the different parts of the brain. Loss of or damage to the myelin sheath—demyelination—plays a major role in several chronic neurological diseases, including Parkinson's disease and multiple sclerosis.

The blood-brain barrier

Glial cells are a critical component of the blood-brain barrier. The BBB was discovered more than a hundred years ago, when curious scientists injected blue dye into the bloodstream of animals. The dye stained every tissue except the brain and spinal column, both of which were somehow able to block absorption of the dye. We now know that the blood-brain barrier is a semipermeable membrane, designed to keep some molecules out of the brain while allowing others in. Toxins that might injure the brain, hormones and neurotransmitters from other parts of the body, and some drugs are kept out, while nutrients and other drugs easily gain access.

The glial cells are essential to the integrity of the BBB. In other parts of the body, molecules can move easily from the tiniest blood vessels (capillaries) into the surrounding tissue through small spaces between the cells of the blood vessel walls. In the brain, glial cells cluster tightly along the capillaries, selectively blocking large molecules from leaving the blood and entering the brain. Recent research suggests that glial cells may be more than mere guardians and housekeepers. They are active players in synapse formation, and dysfunction of glial cells may play a much more important role in the development of neurological disorders like multiple sclerosis than previously thought.

Albert Einstein was one of the greatest scientists of all time—so

brilliant that today his name is synonymous with the word "genius."
Within a few hours of his death in 1955, his brain was removed and
placed in a jar of formaldehyde. Specimens were sent to scientists
around the world for examination. There had been much speculation
about what made Einstein's brain so special. Was his brain bigger? Was
his frontal cortex larger, or did it contain more neurons compared to the
average person? No. In fact, the areas involved in speech and language
were smaller than expected (apparently he didn't speak until he was
four years old). The scientists were confused.

But in the 1980s something unexpected was discovered. Einstein's
brain didn't have more neurons than the non-genius brains it was compared to, but it did have more glial cells, especially in the regions involved
in creativity and complex thinking. It seems likely that we have not yet
begun to understand the many roles glial cells play in the brain, especially in relation to intelligence.

Modern brain imaging techniques

Twenty-first-century technologies are now allowing scientists to study
less obvious and more subtle aspects of brain function, like creativity
and logical thinking. These new methods of investigation rely on the fact
that any area of the brain that is active uses more glucose and oxygen.
These increases can be visualized using several new types of brain scans.
Areas of greater oxygen or glucose consumption light up, while parts
of the brain not actively participating in a particular task remain dark.
Additionally, a new type of quantitative EEG (qEEG) can reveal electrical
activity in various psychological states. Such technologies have begun a
new era of brain mapping, where qualities like mood, creativity, desire
or disgust can be mapped to specific brain regions.

Brain mapping has many applications. Now that we can see into
the living brain, we can image non-depressed brains and compare
them to the brains of depressed individuals to get a more accurate and
specific diagnosis. In turn, this information can help identify the best
treatment options and whether or not they work in a particular individual. Brain mapping is not just of interest to medical science but has

many commercial applications too. In the past decade or so university scientists have begun to collaborate with market researchers to help businesses figure out what pushes our "buy" buttons, and understand not only whether consumers respond to advertising, but *why* they do.

The terms "neuromarketing" and "neuroeconomics" have entered the vocabulary of commerce and academia, adding a whole new dimension to marketing strategies.

Neuromarketing—Messing with our brains?

One well-known story in the world of marketing illustrates just how useful brain mapping is becoming for industry and commerce. In 2008 the fast food company Frito-Lay wanted to increase market share for its snack food Cheetos. These cheesy nibbles, much maligned by nutritionists, were a favourite kids' snack. Frito-Lay wanted to expand into the adult market, so it commissioned a neuromarketing company to find out what would motivate adults to buy more Cheetos. Eating a bag of Cheetos can be a messy business. While most kids don't mind ending up with hands and face smeared with sticky orange goo, Frito-Lay thought this might be a turnoff for adults.

But brain mapping told a different story: the mess was exactly what appealed to adults. Licking the sticky, savoury stuff off their fingers triggered regions of the brain linked to subversion, apparently making them feel like naughty children again. With this information in hand, the company embarked on a series of TV commercials showing adults scoffing Cheetos while engaging in childlike bad behaviour. In one ad, an airline passenger deals with a loudly snoring man in the next seat by sticking two of the worm-like snacks up his nose. In another, a woman in a laundromat takes revenge by adding a bag of the dayglow-orange snacks to a load of someone else's white washing.

Conventional focus groups disliked these commercials, which they thought were mean-spirited. But brain mapping confirmed the earlier work—subconsciously the ads evoked a powerful positive response. So Frito-Lay aired the commercials, bringing in a cool US$47.6 million in increased revenues.

What we learned from the Decade of the Brain

The Decade of the Brain generated more information on the brain's organization and functioning than ever before, but despite the millions of new studies published in a relatively brief period, then and since, and the impressive advances in our ability to spy on living brains, we still know very little about how to keep the brain happy, healthy and working efficiently.

At the same time as knowledge about the brain has exploded, our brains seem to be increasingly fragile. Dementia—the ultimate collapse of the brain and the most feared disease of aging—is a major public health concern. And we have only just begun to uncover the magnitude of the burden of depression in affluent countries around the world.

At the other end of the life span, our children's brains also seem to be more vulnerable to mental health problems: a growing number are being diagnosed with attention deficit and autism spectrum disorders. The economic, social and psychological cost of these conditions is huge. Suicide, which a hundred years ago hardly existed as a major cause of death, is now one of the top ten. Not confined to older adults, it is sadly becoming increasingly common in children and teenagers. The Decade of the Brain made little impact on these statistics.

With all the new technology at our disposal, medical science appears to have no new insights into what causes our neural circuitry to malfunction. Could this be because until now little attention has been paid to the food needs of the brain, to making sure we consume on a daily basis the raw materials our brains need for proper functioning and ongoing maintenance?

CHAPTER 2

Nature versus Nurture

"You," your joys and sorrows, your memories and your ambitions, your sense of personal identity and free will, are in fact no more than the behavior of a vast assembly of nerve cells and their associated molecules.

SIR FRANCIS CRICK,
THE ASTONISHING HYPOTHESIS

Just as in the nineteenth century the twin disciplines of psychology and psychiatry were a natural evolution of our ongoing fascination with the workings of the brain, in the mid-1950s the discipline of cognitive science was the next great advance. Cognitive science brings together researchers from a variety of disciplines. In one laboratory you can find neuroscientists, psychologists, psychiatrists, anthropologists, philosophers, linguists and experts in artificial intelligence all working together.

The common goal of cognitive scientists is to understand the basic brain skills we need to function, and how we acquire them, refine them and prevent them from deterioration. Less concerned with how much we know than with how we learn, cognitive science focuses on how we solve problems, adjust to new challenges and respond emotionally in everyday life. It investigates long- and short-term memory, powers of logic and reasoning, and how well and how fast we can process information that we hear (auditory processing) or see (visual processing)—the very skills that deteriorate with age.

Together, these skill sets make up our intelligence quotient, or IQ. Even in quite small children, exceptional cognitive abilities can be spotted without any formal testing. Preschoolers who are inquisitive, can reason well, solve problems without becoming frustrated, listen and follow instructions have innately good cognition. Once in school, these

25

children thrive and quickly achieve success in basic skills like reading and writing. For these children learning is fast and fun.

But children with poor innate cognition are easily distracted and find it hard to pay attention or remember what they were taught yesterday or last week. For them, school is not such fun. This is, however, where good teaching comes in, because cognitive skills can be taught. They can be improved, often dramatically, with training and patience. Just as weak muscles become stronger with exercise, so innate cognitive abilities can be enhanced, given time and effort. Our brains are infinitely adaptable.

It's all about connections

Although most organs and tissues of the body continually renew themselves, most of the brain's 100 billion neurons are present before birth. A few areas of the brain continue to produce new neurons up to about two years of age. By then, however, the only brain structures that are continually renewing themselves are the hippocampus, the brain region most involved in learning and memory, and responsible for the integration of learning and emotions, and the olfactory bulb located above the nasal cavity, important for the sense of smell. Neurogenesis in these regions continues into old age but steadily declines over the years.[1]

Although newborn brains have more neurons than adult brains, they are much smaller—only about one-quarter the size of an adult brain. Increasing brain size throughout childhood is largely due to changes in the size and complexity of individual neurons, which progressively sprout and extend new dendrites. In about the fifth week after conception, neurons start to form synapses. New synapses appear rapidly up to about two years of age; in an infant's brain, at times as many as forty thousand new synapses are forming per second.[2] Known as blooming, this boisterous period of synapse creation is driven by an infant's eagerness for novelty and stimulation and, most critically, by its interaction with the world around it. In babies and infants reared without physical or social contact, blooming is stunted. The number of synapses formed in the cerebral cortex peaks within the first two to three years of life, and then declines by about one-third between early childhood and adolescence.

This decline is for good reason: while a multitude of synapses creates great potential for learning, a brain with so many possible neuronal pathways is disorganized and slow to respond. Imagine trying to find your way to a new destination using a map where all the possible routes you could take—from highways to side roads and walking paths—are all shown in a jumble of equal interconnections. You would need time to figure out a route, and that route might turn out to be very indirect. So it is with a brain overburdened with surplus synapses. Signals take longer to connect one part of the brain with another, and thinking is slowed. Fortunately, as the brain grows and matures, a process called pruning begins: synapses in underused neuronal pathways are eliminated, while networks reinforced by learning and experience are retained and strengthened.

Blooming and pruning occur at different rates in different brain regions. Areas of the brain involved in sensory input—touch, taste, sight and hearing—grow rapidly in the early postnatal months, whereas brain areas involved in logical thought, planning and reasoning develop steadily up to adolescence. Gradually, the architecture of the brain is shaped, and under ideal conditions an efficient thinking machine is fashioned.

Alcohol consumption and smoking during pregnancy can impair the formation and wiring of fetal brain cells. Similarly, exposure to radiation, infection and some chemicals during the prenatal period can also affect fetal brain development.

Use it or lose it

Not so long ago, it was thought that the ability to make new neural connections—the norm for babies and infants—was lost in older brains. Therefore if a part of the brain became damaged, connectivity between that part of the brain and the functions it controlled was lost forever. We know now that this assumption is wrong. The adult brain is not fixed, but is constantly remodelling itself, continuing to construct new links between neurons in response to experience, and eliminating underused connections. This ability of the brain to change throughout our lifespan is called neuroplasticity.

Changes in the brain can be either positive or negative. Grey matter can expand or shrink. Neurons can extend their dendrites to make new connections, or they can contract, reducing connectivity between different parts of the brain. These physical changes in the brain are mirrored by clear changes in our cognitive abilities. We can become smarter, more empathic and more in tune with the world around us, less anxious and able to think on our feet. Or we can become depressed, isolated and less functional.

Recent work suggests that memories are not just stored in synapses as originally thought. During the learning process, changes occur in the neurons themselves that are probably held in the nucleus of the cell, in its DNA. These changes appear to be permanent, so that provided the brain cells themselves survive, new synapses can be formed and memories retrieved if axons are severed or dendrites shrink.[3] This is good news for anyone who has suffered a stroke or traumatic brain injury.

In his popular 2007 book *The Brain That Changes Itself: Stories of Personal Triumph from the Frontiers of Brain Science*, Canadian psychiatrist Norman Doidge, MD, gives real-life examples of the brain's ability to adapt and change through the creation of new circuitry. This capacity to form and reorganize new synapses is called neuroplasticity. He shows how therapists can tap into this phenomenon to help patients rewire their brains and recover from brain damage caused by trauma or strokes. According to Doidge, neuroplasticity training techniques can help patients overcome depression, anxiety and even learning disabilities.

Anna's story

My friend Anna was a vivacious and vibrant personality. Always sports-minded and a daredevil, she liked nothing better than a physical challenge. She water-skied in summer and went downhill skiing in the winter. On holiday, she was the one who went scuba diving or tried her hand at paragliding or hot-air ballooning. Adventure was in her blood.

As a child, she had very much enjoyed horseback riding, and in her forties she decided to take it up again. On her first day at the stables she was asked to choose a horse. "Don't take the little black mare over there," warned the owner. "She's temperamental and unpredictable." But Anna ignored the advice. "Give her to me. I'll quickly tame her," she insisted. At first all went well. The little black mare seemed to adore Anna and would come running over to greet her as soon as she made an appearance. Then one day when Anna was riding, a nearby car backfired. Startled, the horse reared up on her hind legs and galloped off, throwing Anna to the ground. Anna suffered a severe spinal cord injury that severed the axons and nerve fibres connecting her brain to her lower body. She was quadriplegic.

She spent one year in a rehabilitation hospital, after which she was told she had made all the progress she was ever likely to make. She was still as mentally sharp as ever and could feed herself if someone cut up her food and strapped a spoon into her hand. But for all other functions she was completely dependent on others. The doctors said she would never walk again. Anna would require a wheelchair for the rest of her life.

But now the same headstrong determination that had led her to choose the most unpredictable horse at the stables kicked in. She needed to regain her independence. At home, she started a series of rigorous exercises under the care of a physical therapist. Her first challenge was to get in and out of bed by herself, using her arms and a bed trapeze suspended from the ceiling. She practised the same movement over and over again for days and months until, eventually, she could do it.

Next she worked on reminding the muscles controlling her bladder and rectum how they used to function, willing them to work. After many months of trying, eventually she regained control and was no longer incontinent. Two years after her accident, she could dress and undress, get in and out of bed, and move to and from the kitchen and bathroom without help—huge steps towards independence. Although progress was painstakingly slow, she continued to advance, doing specialized exercises for six to eight hours each and every day.

Five years later, she can walk for up to a mile at a time using only a cane, although she finds it tiring and uses a wheelchair when travelling or shopping. She drives a little sports car specially adapted for her needs and uses it to visit family and friends. Anna insists with a laugh that she would be completely independent if only she could collapse her wheelchair and load it into the trunk of her car by herself. Her remarkable recovery has confounded all medical expectations.

While Anna's determination and perseverance are probably exceptional, her story is a perfect example of the persistence of memories in neurons. With appropriate stimulation, old neural pathways can be reactivated and new ones formed.

Learning and memory

Short-term memory allows us to keep information in our brains for brief periods—seconds rather than minutes—and relies heavily on our ability to pay attention. It is an essential first step in the learning process. Long-term memory is any fact or skill you have learned that is preserved for the future, even if you acquired it only a few moments ago.

Short-term memory mainly involves the prefrontal cortex—the part of the brain located behind the forehead—although other areas are also involved. The prefrontal cortex is responsible for executive function, coordinating the functions of the different parts of the brain and the messages it sends to different parts of the body. It is one of the last regions to reach maturity during brain development and continues to mature well into our twenties. Because short-term memory works through biochemical changes in the brain, it requires the presence of glucose as well as hormones and neurotransmitters like dopamine, noradrenaline, serotonin and acetylcholine.

Once we have acquired new information, we need to store it so that it can be summoned up at a future date. This process involves converting short-term memories into long-term memories and filing them away for later recovery. While short-term memory is temporary, fragile and largely biochemical in nature, converting new information into long-term memory relies on synapse formation as well as repetition and practice to strengthen those synapses. Each time a memory is recalled, whether it's a name, a new skill or an incident, the connections between neurons are reactivated and the synapses are reinforced.

Working memory usually involves a combination of both short- and long-term memory and allows us to juggle multiple pieces of information—either new or retrieved from storage—in our brains while using them. Imagine you receive a long-winded voice mail message with a callback number. After you finish listening, can you still remember the caller's name and phone number, and write them down correctly? If not, your working memory may be poor. Like short-term memory, working memory requires the presence in the brain of neurotransmitters like dopamine and serotonin, and hormones like adrenaline and noradrenaline.[4]

People with poor working memory may have difficulty following multi-step instructions like filling in a complicated form, or they may forget something that was just said in conversation. On the other hand, those with exceptional innate working memory make awesome bridge partners!

Where were you when Kennedy died?

Almost anyone who is old enough remembers where they were and who they were with when they heard that U.S. President John F. Kennedy had been assassinated. And we all probably remember our first kiss with snapshot clarity. A child caught doing something wrong and who experiences a strong sense of shame or embarrassment when confronted will have a lifelong memory of that event, even down to what he was wearing at the time.

Memories formed in the context of very strong emotions, either positive or negative, create a flashbulb image of that moment that is seared into the brain. Such a memory will be easily recalled and is often accompanied by similar emotional sensations to those experienced at the time it was formed. People who have experienced or witnessed a profoundly disturbing event, especially if it involves violence or disaster, can develop post-traumatic stress disorder (PTSD), a debilitating condition that, as we will see in Chapter 6, can be helped by diet and supplements.

Remembering adverse stressful events is important for our survival, tuning us in to situations where we ought to be wary in future. But hypervigilance can have long-term negative consequences for our brains and interfere with cognition and neuroplasticity.

The happy brain

With the growing epidemic of dementia, a major focus of cognitive research is to understand how cognition deteriorates: how and why we lose our memory, judgment and reasoning powers, as well as emotional attachments to friends and family.

Meanwhile, other cognitive scientists are turning their attention to investigating what makes us more social, content and productive—more fulfilled as human beings. One of those is Daniel Gilbert, Harvard psychology professor and author of *Stumbling on Happiness*. He says that the lives lived by our ancestors were nasty, brutish and short. For them, a day's work was to get up in the morning and basically try not to die before bedtime— there was little time to think about personal fulfillment. But today, for those of us lucky to live in the privileged Western world, our principal motivator and the prime driver of human existence is the pursuit of happiness.

We sometimes shy away from discussing or expressing feelings of happiness, either because of a superstitious belief that being happy and showing it will bring bad luck, or because we feel we may be perceived as self-focused and shallow. But Gilbert thinks we need to rethink these attitudes: "I think the problem with the word 'happiness' is that it sounds . . . like something trivial that we shouldn't be concerned with. But just set aside the word and . . . you quickly realize that not only should we be concerned with the study of happiness, but that it's impossible to be concerned with anything else. Pascal says: 'All men seek happiness. This is without exception . . . This is the motive of every action of every man, even of those who hang themselves.' How could the goal of all human behavior be a trivial thing?"[5]

Happiness genes

According to psychologists, happiness consists of at least two distinct parts: hedonia, which generally corresponds to feelings of pleasure, and eudaimonia, which essentially relates to a sense of satisfaction—a life well lived, one that is meaningful and engaging. In constitutionally happy individuals, these two facets of happiness significantly overlap.[6]

Although our understanding of the neurobiology of happiness is only in its infancy, we do know that some individuals find it easier to be happy than others. So are the brains of those who are generally happy genetically different from those who are not? Some evidence suggests that genes do play a significant role. In 2011, the United Nations invited member countries to measure happiness. Samples from each country were asked to rank themselves on a scale of zero to ten, where zero represents the worst and ten the best possible life imaginable. Out of 158 countries ranked in 2015, the ten happiest were Switzerland, Iceland, Denmark, Norway, Canada, Finland, the Netherlands, Sweden, New Zealand and Australia. The United States ranked fifteenth.

Since Denmark regularly tops the charts for the highest levels of reported happiness, researchers examined the genetic makeup in one hundred countries and compared their genes to those of the Danes. The more similar they were to the Danish population, the happier people reported they were. Even when adjusted for many other factors known to affect happiness—affluence, religion, geography and health and social services—genetic makeup seemed to count.

Curious if there was any association between reported levels of happiness and genes linked to mood, the researchers then looked at a mutation in a gene that influences serotonin metabolism. A short version of this gene is linked to higher levels of neuroticism and lower life satisfaction. To their surprise, they found their hypothesis confirmed: the mutation was more common in countries that ranked low on the happiness scale, like Italy. Denmark and the Netherlands had the lowest incidence of this particular gene mutation.

The final surprise was when the researchers matched the reported well-being of Americans with the country of origin of their ancestors. Americans with ancestral links to the happiest countries several generations back reported greater personal happiness.[7]

Brain health and chronic disease

Negative emotional states appear to correlate with poorer overall physical health. Conversely, happiness and what researchers call "emotional vitality" have a positive influence on physical health. Emotional vitality, which is similar to eudaimonia, is defined as "a sense of positive energy, an ability to regulate behaviour and emotions, and a feeling of engagement in life."[8] Those who score high on emotional vitality have good cognitive skills that seem to go hand in hand with good physical health. They have a lower risk of heart disease, stroke and diabetes, and were found to age better.[9] One study has even shown that children who can stay focused on a task and have a generally positive outlook at age seven have better reported general health thirty years later.[10]

Should we be surprised by this link between mental vitality and physical health? Not really. The very same neurotransmitters and hormones that control cognitive skills also regulate the electrical stability of the heart, the operation of the immune system and digestion. And the functioning of those systems depends on the availability of neurotransmitters—the signalling molecules they make. As we will see in later chapters, the generation and activity of those neurotransmitters depends not only on our genetic makeup, but also on how and what we eat.

The empathic brain

A less egocentric cognitive skill, one that recognizes that the happiness of others is just as important as our own, is empathy. Empathy is the ability not only to put ourselves in the shoes of others and recognize their feelings but also to respond appropriately to that recognition. Empathy allows us to identify with both the positive and negative feelings of others, and understand and accept that people may have views different from our own. It is the foundation of a just and tolerant society.

Conversely, lack of empathy is at the root of many social conflicts. It is a hallmark of the psychopath—the unsettling propensity in some members of society for antisocial behaviour and cold-blooded cruelty. Psychopaths are unconcerned by the pain of others. But they don't completely lack empathy. Whereas for most people empathy is the default mode, psychopaths can switch it on and off at will, appearing charming and kind much of the time but capable of callous and sadistic actions at others. Lack of empathy is one factor used in the diagnosis of narcissistic and antisocial personality disorders.

Adults and children with autism spectrum disorder are often thought to be devoid of empathy since they have problems with social interaction and communication. But research suggests that while they may be aware of the feelings of others, they have difficulty interpreting and understanding those feelings.[11]

Mirror neurons

In the prefrontal cortex, there is a population of neurons that fire when we move—reach for our cellphones when they ring, for example. A proportion of these neurons also fire when we watch someone else do the same thing. Similarly, neurons fire when we experience pain or are upset, and a subset of those neurons fire when we watch pain being inflicted on someone else. Discovered in the brains of monkeys by a team of Italian researchers in the 1990s, these neurons mirror the behaviour or emotions of others, as if we ourselves were having the same experience. Hence the name "mirror neurons."

The existence of mirror neurons explains why we are happier when we are surrounded by happy people. If you smile at me, some of the mirror neurons that activate when I smile also fire, and I feel some of the emotions normally associated with smiling. Mirror neurons are essential for social interactions. Without them we would not be able to read the emotions, actions or intentions of the people around us. Some research suggests that reduced or dysfunctional mirror neuron function explains some of the symptoms seen in autism.[12]

I feel your pain

Maddy was an energetic eight-year-old who loved to run. After winning a number of races at her school, she qualified for city and then provincial competitions. Her best friend at school, Jane, was also a runner, and also qualified for the provincial finals. The girls practised intensely. Every night after dinner they could be found running on the track beside the boardwalk, timed by one of their parents. Their anticipation and excitement was intense. They were the first from their school to qualify for these finals for many years.

On the day of the race, Maddy and Jane met up at the competition. But something tragic had happened the night before: Jane's mother, who had been battling cancer for some years, had died. In the midst of all the sorrow and confusion, Jane and her family decided that she should run in the race anyway. She wanted to run; she had practised and practised. The family would come and cheer her on.

Both girls started out well and were comfortably ahead of the pack. But when the race finished there was no sign of either girl. Concerned, their parents went to seek them out and found them halfway along the course. Jane sat sobbing uncontrollably, and Maddy sat with her arm around her, sobbing too. Later, Maddy told her parents how disappointed she was with the outcome of the race. "I so wanted to win," she said afterwards. "But what could I do? I couldn't leave my friend crying."

What was interesting was that Maddy really had no idea why she herself was crying. She simply felt Jane's pain.

Empathy, genes and learning

Somewhere in the left prefrontal cortex lies an "empathy circuit." Most research has shown that we all lie somewhere on an empathy spectrum from low to high. Simon Baron-Cohen, a professor at Cambridge University in the United Kingdom, is an expert in developmental psychopathology. Where we are on that scale depends on the functioning of our empathy circuit, which in turn depends on many factors, from genes to upbringing and cultural environment, he says. Genes linked to neurotransmitter synthesis and metabolism, hormones, and neuronal connectivity in the prefrontal cortex are all thought to play a role.[13]

Other U.K. researchers, at the University of Oxford, have been studying the neurological underpinnings of empathy for some time. Could they identify an area of the brain that controls empathic responses? they wondered. And if so, was it larger or more active in those who displayed the most empathy and generosity? Using brain scanning techniques, they found that a small part of the anterior cingulate cortex—the sub-genual anterior cingulate cortex (sgACC)—is responsible. The ACC is a part of the brain involved in the control of a number of automatic processes, such as blood pressure and heart rate. It is also important for several higher-level functions, including impulse control, decision making and emotions.

When participants in the study were figuring out how they could help others, only the sgACC lit up on brain scans. The researchers also found that their original hunch was correct—the sgACC was larger and more active in those who scored highly on psychological tests of empathy. Even more interesting, the area was not active when the research subjects were learning to carry out a task when they themselves were favoured.[14] Learning that empathy is located in a very specific area of the brain is an important breakthrough. Many psychiatric conditions involve a lack of empathy, and this discovery may help with diagnosis and with the development of new treatments.

Empathy is not just a human trait. Many studies have shown empathy in animals. If the parent of an infant is upset and shows it, not only will the baby cry, but the family dog may also show distress. When research-ers trained monkeys in the 1960s to pull a chain to obtain food, the monkeys ate greedily and made frequent visits to fill up. When they then wired the system so that if the chain was pulled an electric shock was administered to another monkey, the chain was pulled less and less frequently. One monkey went twelve straight days without food rather than knowingly inflict pain on a fellow monkey.

Empathy and mirror neurons

The development of empathy depends not only on fully functioning mirror neurons but also on the role models a child is exposed to—par-ents, teachers and peers. Animal experiments and observational stud-ies in human subjects show the development of empathy depends on the opportunity to form close, caring relationships in infancy. For it to flourish, we need to bond with "special others" from an early age and form attachments that reflect comfort and closeness.

Mirror neurons may also be involved in "copycat" behaviours. These behaviours are the fundamental principle of neuromarketing, discussed in Chapter 1. We see someone eat ice cream in a TV commercial and suddenly we start digging in the freezer for some ourselves. Some scientists are also concerned that the high level of exposure to violence through TV and video games will lead to mirroring behaviour and perhaps ultimately a more violent society. Well-known expert on mirror neurons Dr. Marco Iacoboni, MD, professor of psychiatry at UCLA, is among them. "There is convincing behavioral evidence linking media violence with imitative violence," he says. "Mirror neurons provide a plausible neurobiological mechanism that explains why being exposed to media violence leads to imitative violence."

Abusive or unaffectionate parenting has been linked to a host of aberrant behaviours in later life, such as bullying, substance abuse and juvenile delinquency. Bullying has become a significant problem in our schools. In a 2007 survey of Canadian attitudes toward learning, 38 per cent of adult males and 30 per cent of adult females reported occasional or frequent bullying during their school years.[15] Researchers speculate that bullies know very well what their victims feel; they recognize the pain they are inflicting but either don't care or actually derive pleasure from it.[16] Bullying is not a normal part of growing up and can have severe mental health repercussions. A disturbing number of teenage suicides are linked to school bullying. Bullying in childhood is predictive of violence in adulthood.[17]

Taught or caught?

Since empathy is both innate and learned behaviour, some school programs attempt to increase empathy in young children, especially those who may not have had the best start in life. One pioneering program, started in Toronto by child advocate and former kindergarten teacher Mary Gordon in 1996 and now used worldwide, is called Roots of Empathy. Roots of Empathy is an evidence-based classroom program that has shown dramatic results in improving children's cooperative and kind behaviour to one another and decreasing aggression.[18]

At the start of the school year the program introduces a tiny teacher—a baby two to four months old—into the classroom. Over the year the baby visits the classroom with its mother or father and a specially trained facilitator. The program focuses on the relationship between the parents and the infant. The children learn how to recognize the emotions of the baby and how it sees and reacts to the world. If the baby cries, the children are asked to decide why it's crying.

As the kids watch the baby grow and develop, they learn how to identify the needs and feelings of the baby. By observing the love and care of the parent for the baby, they learn how to mirror that behaviour in their own lives. "There's no empathy app—empathy must be 'caught,' not taught," says Gordon. "They learn how to respect all the baby's different moods, and they learn that caring for the baby—even changing a poopy diaper—is an act of love. They see the humanity in the baby and find it in themselves."

A preposterous hypothesis?

We now spend billions of dollars developing drugs to fix broken brains. We agonize over whether the growing incidence of mental health problems is related to our genetics, the increasingly toxic environment in which we live, the stress of life in overcrowded cities or some other factors as yet undiscovered.

Our brains, in their structure and basic genetics, have not changed in the past million years. They still have the same need for oxygen, water and food. But our diet is another matter. For the bulk of human history, we satisfied our hunger by hunting wild animals and collecting wild plants. Hunter-gatherer diets were generally low in energy and rich in the essential nutrients. But industrialization has transformed modern food so that today it is generally calorie rich and nutrient poor. And clever backroom scientists know how to tweak the taste of cheap, nutritionally worthless foods to tantalize our taste buds, so those same foods have become our foods of choice.

What if the increasing fragility of our children's brains, and the explosive anger of road rage or random mass shootings, were consequences of inadequate modern diets? What if depression were the brain crying out for the vitamins and other essential nutrients it needs to manufacture neurotransmitters like dopamine or serotonin? Suppose that preventing the tragic decline of cognition in old age were simply a matter of changing diets to ensure an optimal supply of the essential nutrients used by the brain for ongoing repair and maintenance?

Are these just fanciful notions akin to Aristotle's belief that the brain was unnecessary or Gall's theory of phrenology? Not according to current medical literature. It is now accepted that far from being an inevitable part of the aging process, dementia is a lifestyle disease, with poor nutrition being a major risk factor.[19] Every day, new evidence is published that underscores the idea that poor nutrition at any stage of life can compromise brain health. It is the cumulative effect over years of failing to meet the nutritional demands of the brain—to sustain its functioning and repair damage—that leads to its final collapse. The cure for dementia and the prevention of Alzheimer's disease therefore lies in the stomach, not in the brain or the medicine cabinet.

Nutritionally oriented physician, prolific author and popular speaker Dr. Emanuel Cheraskin, MD (1916–2001), famously said, "Man is a food dependent creature. Do not feed him and he will die. Feed him improperly and parts of him die." He might well have added "including his brain." In the next two chapters, we will see that the workings of the brain—the behaviour of Sir Francis Crick's "vast assembly of nerve cells and their associated molecules"—depend on a steady supply of an array of nutrients from fats to protein to vitamins and minerals, a fact generally ignored in thinking about brain health.

CHAPTER 3

The Nutrition-Cognition Connection

How can we hope to understand disease if we have no idea why cells work the way they do?

NICK LANE,
The Vital Question: Energy, Evolution,
and the Origins of Complex Life

This is your brain in slow motion

The woman in my waiting room looks tired and dispirited. I discover she is a sociology professor at a local university—her dream job, she says. But it has its problems. Working at a top-notch university means that you have not only to teach but also do research, and that research must be published. As the saying goes, publish or perish.

This professor feels she is on the verge of perishing. She has writer's block and her teaching is also suffering. She can't seem to organize material for her lectures. Faced with a pile of student essays to mark, she doesn't know where to begin. Listless and apathetic, she procrastinates, and the work piles up. Never one to cry easily, suddenly she is bursting into tears at the drop of a hat. Now she can hardly face work at all. "My brain just won't work," she groans. "I think it's ground to a halt."

As she tells me her story, I am looking at the five-day food diary I asked her to complete in advance of her appointment. No breakfast except black coffee, which she drinks throughout the day. She doesn't always stop work for lunch either, though occasionally she has a sandwich or sushi. Dinner is not much better. "I live alone," she explains, "and I don't cook much." So on her way home she might grab another sandwich from the cafeteria, or drop by a local fish and chip shop for some battered and deep-fried fish with french fries.

I ask her if she ever gets hungry. "Not really," she says, "and if I do, I'll have another coffee and smoke a cigarette. Cigarettes and coffee get me through the day."

You can't run a brain on coffee and cigarettes

Caffeine and nicotine are both brain stimulants. In the short term, nicotine can certainly increase alertness, since it opens up blood vessels to increase blood flow to the brain. But in the long term it causes those same blood vessels to narrow, limiting the flow of oxygen, glucose and essential nutrition to the brain. Because of its impact on the health of blood vessels, smoking is a long-term risk factor for heart disease and stroke, as well as dementia and Alzheimer's disease.[1] Apart from nicotine, other chemicals in cigarette smoke can have toxic effects on blood vessels and do similar damage.

Caffeine has been consumed since ancient times in many different forms. Certainly it can increase attention and improve psychomotor skills—those skills that involve both physical and mental activity, like driving a car or playing a musical instrument. Many sports and energy drinks, as well as the ubiquitous colas, owe their popularity to their caffeine content. A little coffee—one or two cups a day—seems to have health benefits, possibly due to coffee's antioxidant effect. Higher caffeine intake might also help reduce the risk of type 2 diabetes. But too much coffee constricts blood vessels and eventually affects learning.[2]

This woman was using coffee and cigarettes to kick-start her brain and keep herself on task at work—giving her brain an occasional shove instead of the steady supply of fuel it needed. This is like getting someone to push your car when it is out of gas. You can get rolling for a while, but the car will inevitably stop again and you'll need another push. Just as a car cannot function without gas no matter how sophisticated its engineering, so even the smartest brain can stall without proper fuel. And that fuel is food.

Oxygen and the brain

As the most metabolically active organ of the body, the brain has especially high needs for nutrients. These are the raw materials needed to create and maintain the brain's structural integrity, build and repair the neurons' myelin sheath, protect the brain from damage caused by stress or overuse, and heal it if it is injured.

Oxygen is the brain's most basic requirement for survival, needed to generate energy. At the heart of this energy production are small but fascinating structures inside cells: the mitochondria. Mitochondria produce the energy that cells need to function and in the process generate free radicals that can wreak havoc in cells when left unchecked (more about free radicals in Chapter 4). Also known as the powerhouses of cells, these tiny structures look very like cells themselves—a cell within a cell, so to speak. They even have their own DNA. And without a steady supply of oxygen, the mitochondria simply can't function.

Many billions of years ago, mitochondria may have been free-living bacteria. Bacteria were here on Earth first, before plants or animals, and can survive the harshest of environments; some species can even feed on concrete and survive the superheated waters of hot springs. Biologists believe that a freak accident may have allowed one bacterium to take up residence inside another. The infecting bacterium would have generated extra energy for the host cell, which would have allowed the pairing to thrive and increase in biological complexity—a possible driver for evolution. Many lines of evidence now support this theory. Mitochondria are not free-living organisms any more, however. They now depend on the host cell to provide key nutrients they themselves need to survive.

The number of mitochondria varies from cell to cell. Red cells have none, whereas liver cells may each have up to two thousand. In heart muscle, where energy needs are high, 40 per cent of the cell's cytoplasm is composed of mitochondria. These critical organelles are dynamic—frequently shifting around in cells to deliver energy where it is needed.

In neurons, for example, mitochondria will travel along the length of the axons to deliver energy at the synapse.

Chapter 4 will explore how the very survival of mitochondria depends on them being properly fed.

Our sugar-seeking brains

Like all the cells in our body, brain cells depend on a steady supply of glucose. This glucose comes from many sources. It occurs naturally in all plant-based foods, not just those that taste sweet, like fruit. In plants that don't taste sweet, like wheat or rice, the sugar is in the form of starch, which consists of multiple glucose molecules linked together into long chains. Starch is the way plants store energy for later use. It doesn't taste sweet because it is not a sugar, not yet anyway, so it doesn't stimulate the sweet-sensing taste buds on our tongues. But don't be deceived. As soon as our digestive enzymes get to work on it, most starch rapidly becomes sugar and enters the bloodstream. Consider starch as sugar in disguise.

Our brain's relationship with sugar is complicated. Glucose in the blood triggers the release of insulin, which in turn prompts cells either to use the glucose for energy or store the excess in muscle and liver cells as glycogen. Glycogen is our emergency sugar supply. We use it for sudden bursts of energy, like fleeing from a tiger or running for a bus. However, our muscles and liver have a very limited storage capacity for glycogen, and when those stores are replete, excess circulating sugar is stored as fat.

If we go too long without food, the brain signals the pancreas to make another hormone, glucagon. Glucagon triggers fat stores to release stored sugar. Insulin and glucagon work in tandem to ensure that even if energy intake fluctuates, all cells, including brain cells, receive the glucose they need to function.

Pushing the panic button

The health of all cells depends on a steady supply of glucose for energy, and insulin, secreted by the pancreas, is needed to get the glucose into cells. Insulin works by attaching itself to a molecule on a cell's surface—the insulin receptor—which unlocks cells and allows the passage of glucose inside. "Open up," says the insulin, and the cells gratefully oblige. When more glucose is available than the cells need for energy, the excess will be stored as fat for future use.

But provoking spikes of insulin through high sugar intakes means that circulating blood levels of glucose drop, since insulin causes the glucose to be removed into storage. Now the brain panics. It simply can't function without sugar. "Please get me more sugar—another cookie, a piece of bread, a glass of orange juice," it demands. "Anything with sugar or starch will do." If we give in to these demands with more of the same types of food a vicious cycle begins: blood sugar spikes again, followed by a spike in insulin, followed by another drop in blood glucose and a desire for more sugar. Now we are on a rollercoaster of sugar highs and lows, and, in all likelihood, firmly on the road to weight gain.

Any type of sugar, whether naturally occurring, as in fruit juice, or added, as in a can of cola, can cause a sugar spike which in turn provokes a spike of insulin. Starchy foods can cause a similar insulin spike, especially if they are in the form of highly processed grains. These are grains that have been finely ground into flour and made into crackers or bread. Pulverizing grains allows digestive enzymes easy access to the starch, which means they are quickly converted to glucose, and blood sugar rises fast.

The glycemic index (GI) ranks foods on a scale from 1 to 100 based on how fast and how high they raise blood sugar, with 100 representing the blood sugar impact of 50 g of glucose. On this scale, a slice of white baguette bread has a GI of 95—almost as high as pure glucose. A slice of pizza with tomato sauce and Parmesan cheese comes in at 80, and a fruit roll-up, often considered a heathy addition to a child's lunch box, comes in at 99.[3] Foods that raise blood glucose too fast and too high are called high glycemic foods.

Developing resistance

Over time, excessive amounts of insulin can cause "insulin resistance." Overwhelmed by insulin, cells ignore insulin's demand to "open up" and allow sugar inside. They do this by removing the insulin receptors from their cell surface so that glucose cannot enter. But insulin's job is not restricted to taking sugar out of the bloodstream and feeding it to cells. Insulin is our main storage hormone, needed to store other nutrients. If cells become deaf to insulin's command, we cannot get any nutrients into cells—the amino acids needed to make hormones or neurotransmitters, and the vitamins and minerals necessary for their manufacture.

Insulin resistance also forces the pancreas to make more and more insulin in an attempt to get sugar out of the blood and into cells. Repeatedly challenging the pancreas to secrete insulin eventually leads to its exhaustion and to type 2 diabetes. Type 2 diabetes can damage the brain and is therefore a major risk factor for dementia. In patients with repeated episodes of low blood sugar, which as we have seen can be caused by too much sugar, detrimental changes have been noted in both the white and grey matter regions of the brain.[4]

Food for thought

The chemical messengers of brain cells, neurotransmitters, dictate every aspect of brain function. They shape memories, control moods, help us sleep soundly and regulate how energetic we feel. Dietary protein is indispensable for the manufacture of many critical neurotransmitters. When we eat protein, our digestive system breaks it down into its basic building blocks—amino acids. Sometimes called the building blocks of life because they are needed to make DNA, amino acids are also the primary constituents of muscles, bones, skin, nails and hair. Some amino acids are essential, meaning we must get them from food; others we can manufacture ourselves.

Our bodies can't store protein, and within one to three days of not meeting our daily requirement we turn to our own muscle fibres to supply the amino acids we depend on to make hormones and neurotransmitters. This damages not only skeletal muscle, but also muscular organs like the heart and kidneys. Recent studies suggest that we have underestimated our need for protein and that the amount we need is significantly higher than current recommendations.[5] But don't eat it all at one meal. The healthiest and most efficient way to consume protein is spread out throughout the day: 25–30 g of protein at breakfast, lunch and dinner works best for most adults.[6] Unfortunately, many people eat their entire daily allowance at one meal, usually dinner.

Protein needs are dependent on age, our level of exercise or exertion, and our state of health. We need more protein if we regularly do vigorous exercise or our job involves heavy physical labour. And when we are sick and don't feel like eating, we continue to need protein. How much we need for optimal health we will also explore in later chapters.

Just-in-time delivery

Like protein, the body can't store neurotransmitters—they must be made lickety-split as needed. In industry, the term "just-in-time inventory" is frequently used. This is an efficiency measure where products are manufactured on demand rather than stockpiled. The components are stored, but the finished products, whether washing machines or tractors, are built only as the orders come in. The body uses the same system to manufacture neurotransmitters. So for the brain to work efficiently, the components we use to make these chemical messengers need to be circulating in our blood at all times, ready for assembly.

Our ability to make neurotransmitters doesn't just depend on what we eat, but also when we eat. We are using up neurotransmitters all the time, so we need to be regularly stocking up on their precursors so that they can be replaced. Remarkable as it may seem, whether or not we can make the right brain chemistry to focus, concentrate or sleep depends not on how we ate yesterday or the day before, but on how we ate at our last meal.[7]

The two major neurotransmitters our professor's brain was likely to be short of are dopamine, a natural antidepressant, and serotonin, needed to calm the brain, screen out distractions and dampen anxiety. Serotonin is especially important later in the day to prevent "busy brain syndrome"—a state of mental unease we experience when we can't seem to let go of the day's preoccupations, and events and thoughts race endlessly and unproductively around in our heads. We also need supplies of serotonin towards the end of the day to make melatonin, needed for deep refreshing sleep. Lack of serotonin is a major cause of insomnia.

No wonder she felt her brain had ground to a halt. Brains can't work efficiently if they are randomly fed. And she wasn't just eating randomly. She was hardly eating at all.

Dopamine, serotonin and diet

The building block for dopamine is a non-essential amino acid, tyrosine. It is not essential because we can manufacture it from another amino acid, phenylalanine. However, tyrosine is in high demand because it is needed to make a number of other critical chemicals, including the stress hormones adrenaline and noradrenaline. Tyrosine is also the precursor for the endorphins, the body's natural painkillers and feel-good hormones, and for coenzyme Q10 (CoQ10), also known as ubiquinone. Ubiquinone performs two important functions. Along with oxygen, mitochondria need it to produce energy. It also acts as a powerful antioxidant, protecting cells against damage caused by the harmful molecules called free radicals.

Tyrosine is required to manufacture two other very important chemicals in the body: the thyroid hormone thyroxin, and melanin, the pigment of skin and hair. With such a huge to-do list, we could easily run out of tyrosine, especially if we eat a low-protein diet. Mood, intellectual and physical performance, and sensitivity to pain are all altered by low dietary tyrosine intake.[8]

The basic building block for serotonin is another amino acid—tryptophan—which *is* essential. Unlike tyrosine, which is the most abundant amino acid in protein-rich food, tryptophan is the least plentiful, and many protein-rich foods contain very little. Serotonin is highly concentrated in key areas of the brain collectively known as our "social brain." The social brain regulates decision making and social interactions. Experimentally, depleting the brain of serotonin has serious consequences, increasing aggression, impulsivity, anxiety and depression.[9]

Poor eating habits affect our ability to make dopamine and serotonin, and this is made worse by physical and emotional stress, lack of exercise, and high intakes of caffeine and alcohol. But with careful attention to what and when we eat, we can modify brain function to serve us better. It is possible to optimize dopamine when we need to be alert, focused and energetic, and to raise serotonin in the evening, helping us to let go of the concerns of the day and sleep like a baby. We will explore how in later chapters.

The playwright and the actress

Famous Irish playwright and Nobel Prize winner George Bernard Shaw was not one to suffer fools gladly and was known for his sometimes brutal putdowns. The story goes that he was at a party where he got into conversation with an actress. The actress was on a diet and refused to eat because she was afraid of getting fat. Shaw was skeptical. "No diet will remove all the fat from your body," he cautioned. "The brain is entirely fat. Without a brain, you might look good, but all you could do is run for public office." (It seems he reserved some of his harshest barbs for politicians!)

Shaw was right about the brain. It *is* mostly fat—around 60 per cent— but it needs to be the right sort of fat. Brain cells require very specialized fats, called omega-3 and omega-6 fatty acids. These are polyunsaturated fatty acids (PUFAs). Both fats are partners in the prevention of many chronic diseases associated with aging, like heart disease and dementia. Both are also essential, meaning we cannot manufacture them and must get them from food. PUFAs are critical for proper brain growth and development, as well as lifelong brain health.[10]

Although omega-6 fats are essential, a high intake can promote inflammation. Inflammation is usually thought of as a bad thing, although it plays a necessary role in the immune system's response to infection and is crucial for proper wound healing. But persistent inflammation is believed to be at the root of many degenerative diseases—not only heart disease and arthritis, but also brain-damaging conditions like multiple sclerosis, Parkinson's and Alzheimer's disease.

Omega-3 fats, on the other hand, are anti-inflammatory. Found in fatty fish like salmon, sardines and other seafood, and some plants and nut oils, they are normal constituents of the membranes of all cells, including brain cells. Within the family of omega-3 fats are two well-studied members, the long-chain fatty acids eicosapentaenoic acid (EPA) and docosahexaenoic acid (DHA). Found mainly in marine sources like fatty fish, they are not present in plant sources of omega-3 fats, like flaxseed oil or canola.

Together, EPA and DHA control the ability of neurons to manufacture serotonin and release it into the synapse. Low blood levels of EPA and DHA are common in a wide range of psychiatric disorders associated with serotonin dysregulation, including attention deficit hyperactivity disorder, bipolar disorder, schizophrenia and dementia.[11]

A matter of balance

Evidence suggests that humans evolved consuming a ratio of omega-6 to omega-3 fats of approximately 1:1. This balance regulated the body's inflammatory responses perfectly, allowing the necessary rise in inflammation for the purposes of healing or fighting infection, but preventing the development of the persistent inflammation that causes tissue damage. Modern diets are deficient in omega-3 fats and have excessive amounts of omega-6s, so today the balance is more likely to be 15:1 to 20:1. This is a three- to fourfold increase in the ratio from a hundred years ago.

While diets rich in omega-3 fatty acids are gaining appreciation for their role in supporting cognitive function, diets that are high in two other fats—saturated fats and trans fats—can harm the brain. Saturated fats occur in dairy foods like butter, cream and cheese, in egg yolks, and in the fat of animals, especially in meat from beef cattle reared in feedlots and fed corn and other grains. Grass-fed beef, on the other hand, has a fat profile similar to salmon: it is higher in omega-3 fats and lower in saturated fats.

Whereas PUFAs are needed to give fluidity and flexibility to cell membranes, saturated fats provide structure and support, and are integral to the organization of the cell. However, saturated fats are not essential. We make them ourselves. In fact, any excess calories we consume eventually get converted into saturated fat. Shaw was right. You can't have a body without fat, and that includes saturated fat.

Seeing what we want to see

Since the 1980s we have been taught that saturated fats and the cholesterol in food were the root cause of heart disease, and a low-fat, low-cholesterol diet has been the cornerstone of public health advice. But thirty-five years later that advice is about to be overturned. The advisory committee for the U.S. dietary guidelines has suggested abandoning recommendations to strictly limit intake of cholesterol, saturated fat and total fat. The research that initially appeared to support the idea that saturated fat was the cause of heart disease was inadequate to begin with and not confirmed by subsequent studies.[12] Reproducibility, you'll remember, is one of the hallmarks of reliable research. Indeed, study after study has shown no links between cardiovascular disease and intake of cholesterol-rich foods like eggs or saturated fats like butter.[13]

The original research that started the low-fat craze was done by a doctor called Ancel Keys. Starting in the 1950s, he published research from seven countries showing that the higher the percentage of calories consumed as fat, the greater the risk of death from heart disease. Although data was actually available from twenty-two countries, Keys excluded data from sixteen of them. At the time some researchers questioned this choice, pointing out that if all twenty-two countries were analyzed together, the association no longer held.[14]

Like Franz Joseph Gall and his theory of phrenology, Keys appears to have disregarded data that didn't fit his hypothesis. And like the theory of phrenology, the fat/cholesterol hypothesis became so firmly ingrained in the public consciousness that it would take many decades before it was re-examined. Thankfully that day is here. It's now okay to put butter on your vegetables or have an egg for breakfast—you won't keel over from a heart attack! In later chapters we will see that avoiding eggs, particularly egg yolks, may have a detrimental impact on memory, particularly during pregnancy and in old age.

So, can we now eat as much saturated fat as we like? Not really. At least in animal studies, a high intake of saturated fat can interfere with dopamine function.[15] Saturated fat is also high in calories, so a little goes a long way. And we would be wise to remember the lessons about saturated fat from weight-loss studies. A decade or two ago the Atkins diet for weight loss received a lot of publicity. The Atkins diet severely restricts sugars and starch, even those from natural sources like fruits and vegetables, while allowing unlimited amounts of protein and fat, including food high in saturated fat like eggs, bacon and sausages.

Heart specialists were horrified when this diet became popular. Then studies began to show that not only was it an effective strategy for weight loss, but it also reduced high triglycerides and cholesterol levels—major risk factors for heart disease.[16] More thorough investigations showed that the Atkins diet increased an undesirable protein in blood called C-reactive protein.[17] CRP levels had not been examined in previous clinical trials.

As a sign of increased circulating inflammation, high CRP not only increases the risk for heart disease, but also affects mental health. Elevated CRP has been linked to increased risk of anxiety and depression, and even dementia. Long-term studies suggest that CRP starts to climb long before clinical signs of dementia appear.[18]

So the message is clear. For several reasons, not the least of which are its high caloric content and potentially damaging effect on the brain, too much saturated fat is bad for us.

Just because it's edible doesn't make it food

On a plane heading to a meeting in Vancouver, my eye is caught by one of the bright and cheerful brochures in the seat pocket in front of me titled "Edibles and Entertainment." It lists the meals, snacks, movies and TV programs available en route. I have to smile. Much as I would like to think that the airline actually understands the distinction between food that nourishes the body, and stuff that is edible and satisfies hunger but has little or no nutritional value, I somehow doubt it. When the food cart comes around, it is laden with high-calorie junk foods that scream added sugar and trans fats.

Trans fats are artificial, man-made fats found mainly in processed foods. They are formed when liquid vegetable oils high in PUFAs are made solid by exposing them to hydrogen at high pressures and temperatures (hydrogenation). From the perspective of the food industry, there are good reasons to modify fats this way. When exposed to excess heat and light, both the omega-6 and omega-3 fatty acids spoil easily and develop an "off" flavour. Trans fats improve the taste and texture of food and extend shelf life. Until recently, they were the darlings of the food industry.

Up to the 1990s, few studies had examined these artificial fats and whether they might be harmful to health. Natural saturated fats like coconut oil, egg yolks, butter and cream had to shoulder the blame, incorrectly as it turned out, for health problems caused by high-fat diets. But trans fats raise LDL cholesterol—the so-called bad cholesterol—and lower HDL cholesterol, the good stuff. They do not behave in the brain like natural fats do; they lower serotonin levels and increase inflammation. Trans fats have been linked to mood disorders and aggressive behaviour.

It is becoming clear that trans fats can interfere with memory at any age. In children, they can integrate into brain cells, commandeering sites in cell membranes that should be occupied by the essential omega-3 and omega-6 fats. Consequently, children who eat a steady diet of fast foods are likely to have compromised brain function. A study from the University of California, San Diego recently linked a higher intake of trans fats in men in their forties—prime earning years when brains need to be in peak condition—to deteriorating memory function.[19] These are fats you definitely don't want in your diet. Some countries, like Denmark, have already successfully eliminated man-made trans fats from food, while others have restricted the amount permissible. But even though they are no longer considered safe, the food industry is fighting to preserve their use in a wide variety of packaged foods.[20]

If you value your brain, start reading labels, ask questions, and resist the store-bought pie crust, frozen pizza, creamers, frosting, microwave popcorn, chips and other snack foods laced with these brain breakers. In further chapters of this book we'll explore the other nutritional needs of the brain as it develops, grows, learns and prospers, and learn how to ensure that it's properly fed at every age.

CHAPTER 4

Vitamins, Minerals and Brain Function

I know of nothing so potent in maintaining good health in laboratory animals as perfectly constituted food; I know nothing so potent in producing ill-health as improperly constituted food. This, too, is the experience of stockbreeders. Is man an exception to a rule so universally applicable to the higher animals?

SIR ROBERT McCARRISON, MD

At the beginning of the twentieth century, nutrition as a serious science was in its infancy and focused primarily on fats, protein and carbohydrates. A balance of these three with a couple of added minerals like calcium and iron was considered a complete diet—all we needed for full and efficient physiological functioning. There was only one problem: laboratory animals fed similar diets got sick and died.

Initially the researchers dismissed these unexpected results. Perhaps it had nothing to do with the food itself. Maybe the diets were just boring—so unpalatable that the animals lost interest in eating, became malnourished and died. But gradually it became clear that fats, proteins and carbohydrates were not enough by themselves for survival and that other, previously unknown, substances were also needed. These were missing from the laboratory-constructed diets.

At first these extra elements were simply called "accessory food factors," but eventually they became known as vitamins, their name emphasizing how vital they were for survival.

How did we miss them?

Vitamins had been overlooked for years because they are present in food only in tiny amounts. Nevertheless, they regulate billions of chemical reactions. They are the catalysts that drive the chemistry of tissues and cells.

They control whether cells live or die, how and if they communicate with one another, and whether they produce needed bioactive molecules like hormones or neurotransmitters. Without vitamins, cellular tasks needed for our very existence slow down and eventually simply grind to a halt. Vitamins are needed for the production of energy and for the immune system to work. In their absence, blood will not clot, wounds cannot heal, and bones and teeth crumble. They are needed to help us see in the dark and to keep us sane.

Although it makes for fascinating reading, it is beyond the scope of this book to give a full account of the flurry of research activity that led to the discovery of vitamins in the early twentieth century. For that story I recommend two excellent books published at the height of medical excitement about vitamins and their impact on health. Both give excellent insights into the work of the many biochemists and physiologists who isolated and purified the accessory food factors in their laboratories, showed that they were essential and established the minimums needed for survival.[1]

Fat soluble and water soluble

Vitamins are grouped into two categories, depending on whether they dissolve in water or in fat. The water-soluble vitamins include the B vitamins and vitamin C.

The B vitamins are chemically unrelated, but since they are found together in nature and work cooperatively with each other, they are all included in one umbrella group. The complex of B vitamins includes vitamin B1 (thiamine), vitamin B2 (riboflavin), vitamin B3 (niacin or nicotinic acid), vitamin B5 (pantothenic acid), vitamin B6 (pyridoxine), biotin, folic acid and B12 (cobalamin). The numbering reflects the order in which they were discovered. Some of the B vitamins are numbered, while some are known mainly by their chemical names.

The remainder of the vitamins are fat soluble: vitamins A, D, E and K. The fat-soluble vitamins are usually found in fatty foods and need to be eaten with fat for proper absorption. Because they are fat soluble, we can store them in fatty tissues like the liver, so it is not so important to get them each and every day. The water-soluble vitamins, on the other hand, leach easily from the body in sweat, urine and other secretions, so they need to be replenished daily. They are also depleted by commonly used medications, especially drugs like diuretics—the so-called water pills.

Water pills are used to treat high blood pressure and remove excess fluid that may have accumulated inappropriately in tissue. They do this by increasing the kidney's output of urine and sodium. But diuretics don't remove just excess fluid and sodium, but also water-soluble nutrients—the B vitamins and vitamin C. And since all the minerals are water soluble, diuretics deplete these essential nutrients too.

Vitamins and brain health

Throughout this book, we will be looking at evidence that the development of the brain, its day-to-day performance, and its maintenance and repair can be compromised by shortages of any of the essential nutrients. But here I want to give a couple of illustrations to show that early research, although almost universally ignored by medicine today, is highly relevant to the health of the brain.

In 1937 the first scientific paper was published revealing that a disease known as pellagra was due not to infection as previously believed, but to a deficiency of one of the B vitamins—niacin or vitamin B3. Clinically, pellagra has three characteristic symptoms, known as the three Ds: diarrhea, dermatitis and dementia. Sadly, if the deficiency continues for long enough, a fourth D, death, becomes inevitable. Pellagra had been observed for at least two hundred years, but until the 1930s nobody knew what caused it.

Niacin is needed to convert carbohydrates into glucose, to metabolize fats and proteins, and to make sex hormones. It is critically important for the nervous system. Because we need it to make adrenal hormones, we use more niacin when we are under stress. If dietary intake is too low we *can* make some niacin ourselves—we make it from tryptophan, the amino acid we also use to make serotonin. But the conversion of trypto-phan to niacin is an extremely wasteful process: it takes approximately sixty milligrams of tryptophan to make a single milligram of niacin.

Is it possible that when our diets are short of niacin, we use up our dietary tryptophan to make it, and therefore have little left over to make serotonin? And could this in turn lead to deterioration in mood and decline of brain function?

Niacin, cholesterol and mood

Wendy was a woman in her fifties. When she first came to me, her main concern was her cholesterol, which had been gradually rising as she went through menopause. Her routine blood tests showed that her LDL cholesterol—the bad stuff—was too high, while her HDL, or good cho-lesterol, was too low. Because she had previously had a bad reaction to statin drugs—the first-line medications used to lower circulating cholesterol levels—she wanted to try modifying her diet instead to see if she could get cholesterol back under control. She had already made some dietary changes herself. She scrupulously avoided all dietary fat. No eggs, only skim milk, fat-free cottage cheese and yogurt. No butter. None of the changes had helped so far.

Since she had tried the low-fat approach, I suggested she give a low-carbohydrate diet a chance. Although controversial, a study had shown that reducing carbohydrate was more effective than a low-fat diet at reducing cholesterol.[2] I explained to Wendy that there was a lot of confusion about what a low-carb diet actually is. I didn't want her to cut back on vegetables and fruit—carbohydrates that are packed full of healthy phytochemicals. Instead, she should avoid sources of added sugar like cookies and candies, and reduce her intake of the starchy carbohydrates—bread, potatoes, pasta and rice, especially in their most processed forms, like bread or crackers—to one serving per meal.

I also suggested she start taking niacin, which increases HDL cholesterol. Many clients don't like taking niacin, because at the doses shown to increase HDL most experience skin flushing. Although this flush is harmless, many people dislike it. (Another form of niacin is marketed as non-flushing, but it does not have the same impact on HDL cholesterol and I don't recommend it.) I do recommend that patients check with their doctors before trying niacin, since some preparations of niacin, especially time-released forms, might adversely affect liver health. Five months later Wendy's doctor tested her cholesterol. To her delight her results looked normal. Her LDL cholesterol had come down into the normal range, and her HDL cholesterol had increased. I suggested she no longer needed to take niacin, and so she stopped.

A year or so later Wendy was in my office. I asked her how she was feeling, and she said she was fine now but she had been depressed. Her mood change seemed to coincide with stopping niacin, so she went back on it and the depression resolved. Since her liver functions were normal, her doctor agreed that it was fine for her to remain on high-dose niacin long term. Her depression has not returned.

The well-fed mitochondrion

Mitochondria need niacin to support their work producing energy. When insufficient niacin is available, that work is compromised. Diminished energy production starts a toxic process of mitochondrial decay—a downward spiral of events where sluggish energy production and a reduced ability of cells to disarm dangerous free radicals first causes the mitochondria to die and eventually leads to the death of cells. Mitochondrial decay is thought to play a central role in Parkinson's disease, multiple sclerosis and dementia.[3]

Try to imagine mitochondria that are properly fed, speeding like bullet trains down the axons of neurons, efficiently shuttling energy down to synapses—just what's needed for neurons to communicate effectively. Now imagine a brain deprived of niacin. At first any available tryptophan in the diet will be used to make niacin, a short-term fix. But if the niacin deficiency persists, tryptophan will be used up and unavailable to make serotonin. Now the typical symptoms of low brain serotonin—anxiety and depression, increased impulsivity and aggression—start to appear.

As the deficiency continues for months or even years, the ability of the mitochondria to produce energy declines. With insufficient energy available, the axons themselves die back, interfering with communication both between different regions of the brain and between the brain and distant parts of the body. It would not be surprising if this neurological slowdown led eventually to the sluggish movement, difficulty communicating, and disorientation in time and space that are the hallmarks of the advanced stages of Alzheimer's disease.

But we mustn't run away with the idea that mitochondrial decay is due entirely to niacin deficiency. As we will see throughout this book, all the essential nutrients are needed for the brain to function, and all are involved either directly or indirectly in maintaining the health of mitochondria.

Recognizing signs and symptoms of deficiency

Once vitamins and minerals were known to be essential—just before the beginning of World War Two—researchers could focus on identifying the diseases that developed when animals were deprived of them. Without iron, we could not make enough hemoglobin to carry oxygen around in our blood and we became anemic. Lack of vitamin C produced a condition called scurvy.

The menace of scurvy had been familiar to seafarers and explorers since ancient times. Although described by Hippocrates, the first detailed accounts are found in the writings of thirteenth-century physicians who accompanied the crusaders on their expeditions. In its early stages the symptoms of scurvy are not very specific—mainly extreme fatigue and irritability—and are easily missed. If the deficiency persists, joints and muscles start to hurt. Severe symptoms develop only after body stores of vitamin C have run out, which takes about three months. Then skin changes become obvious. Purplishblack bruises—ecchymoses—appear on arms and legs, caused by the leakage of blood into the skin. Hair breaks off easily. New hairs may be twisted like little corkscrews.

In the end, spontaneous bleeding, fever and convulsions cause death.

Can you be short of a vitamin without being deficient?

Today we assume that scurvy is no longer a problem, since most people have access to a variety of fruits and vegetables—vitamin-C-rich foods. Certain groups, like pregnant women and the elderly, are known to be vulnerable, especially if they eat limited diets. Alcohol and smoking also deplete vitamin C and increase needs.

Technically, it is impossible to be deficient in any essential nutrient and still be alive, since in all cases extreme deficiency causes death. But not having enough of any one of them to provide optimal metabolic support is malnutrition. The Food and Agricultural Organization of the United Nations (FAO) defines malnutrition as "a pathological condition, brought about by inadequacy of one or more of the nutrients essential for survival, growth, reproduction and the capacity to learn and function in society. It can be mild, moderate or severe, depending on the level of deficiency."

In this context, "nutrients" refers to any of the essentials: vitamins, minerals, essential fats and sufficient protein to provide optimal amounts of all the essential amino acids.

Repairing daily wear and tear

Vitamin C is needed to make collagen, the most abundant molecule in the body after water. Derived from the Greek word for glue, *kolla,* collagen literally holds us together, providing structural support, strength and elasticity for tendons and ligaments, bone, muscles, skin and all internal organs. The visible signs of scurvy—the bleeding and bruising— are due to the fragility of blood vessels, which rupture easily. Collagen is needed for wounds to heal and for the proper formation of scars.

Our bodies need to continually manufacture collagen to repair and maintain body structures damaged by daily wear and tear. This requires a steady supply of vitamin C, which itself is destroyed during collagen production. While scurvy—the most extreme and fatal form of vitamin C deficiency—may not be common, modern diets clearly do not support optimal collagen production. Connective tissue disorders are rampant, and poor-quality collagen or unreliable replacement has been linked to many of them, including osteoporosis, cartilage and disc deterioration, heart murmurs, aneurysms, rotator cuff injuries and hernias.

American Hungarian biochemist Albert Szent-Györgyi was awarded the 1937 Nobel Prize for Physiology or Medicine for the synthesis of vitamin C (or ascorbic acid, to give it its chemical name). In his acceptance speech, he chided the medical profession for oversimplifying the role of vitamin C in health: "The medical profession took a very narrow and very wrong view. Lack of ascorbic acid caused scurvy, so if there was no scurvy there was no lack of ascorbic acid—nothing could be clearer than this. The only trouble was that scurvy is not a first symptom of a lack but a final collapse, a pre-mortal syndrome, and there is a very wide gap between scurvy and full health."

This shadowy region between frank illness and full health is where many people spend the best years of their lives—years when they should be at their peak earning and reproductive capacity and full of vitality. Instead they are tired, listless and irritable. Having postponed childbearing to focus on careers, they may then have difficulty conceiving. It is unfortunate that medical schools no longer train doctors to recognize the signs and symptoms of vitamin deficiencies, so that today scurvy is sometimes missed in the clinic even when the classic signs and symptoms are obvious.[4] Szent-Györgyi would not be surprised.

Vitamin C and the brain

Vitamin C is critical for brain health—even before we are born it plays a central role in brain development. Vitamin C is needed for the manufacture of neurotransmitters like serotonin and dopamine, and to make stress hormones like adrenaline, so it is used up faster under stressful conditions. A study of hospitalized patients, for example, showed that extra vitamin C twice a day helped them cope better with the ordeal of being ill and was associated with a 71 per cent reduction in mood disturbances and a 51 per cent reduction in feelings of distress.[5]

Vitamin C also acts as an antioxidant, protecting the delicate tissues of the brain against free radical attack. Free radicals are missing an electron in their outer shell. Because of this they are highly reactive and unstable, and attempt to stabilize themselves by stealing electrons from other nearby molecules. When these molecules are robbed of electrons they in turn become unstable, and so more free radicals are born. This chain reaction, once begun, can result in extensive and ongoing tissue damage.

Free radicals are generated by our bodies during normal metabolic processes such as the production of energy by mitochondria—simply breathing and digesting our food generates them. Indeed, free radicals are needed for the killing and disposal of bacteria. It is excessive production that's the problem. Smoking, exercise, stress, environmental pollution, surgery and infection increase circulating levels of free radicals. Many commonly used pharmaceutical drugs also increase free radical production.

Because our brains are so metabolically active, our neurons and glial cells are exposed to constant free radical bombardment. Left uncontrolled, this can cause chronic brain inflammation and irreparable damage. One of vitamin C's roles is to convert free radicals into relatively harmless compounds. Other vitamins like vitamin A and vitamin E are also antioxidants. We will discuss these in later chapters.

Minerals are essential too

The discovery that many minerals were also essential was not so dramatic and took place over a longer period. Minerals are found naturally in the earth and oceans, and in every living organism, where they control vital chemical and electrical processes. They are needed to activate enzymes and work in concert with the vitamins.

Some minerals are required in relatively large amounts, and therefore known as macrominerals. These include calcium, phosphorus, potassium, magnesium, sulphur, sodium and chlorine. There are also minor or "trace" minerals that are just as essential but needed in smaller amounts. Trace minerals include iron, copper, zinc, iodine, selenium, cobalt, manganese, molybdenum and bromine. Like vitamins C and E, some minerals can act as antioxidants, including selenium, manganese and zinc. The antioxidant vitamins and minerals work synergistically to protect tissues against free radical tissue damage.

Traditionally, eating plants grown in nutrient-rich soils provided us with minerals. However, mineral-rich agricultural land is increasingly rare as modern farming techniques have depleted minerals by growing crops year after year in the same soil. Crops themselves need certain minerals to grow, so man-made fertilizers are routinely used. These fertilizers provide only the bare minimum needed by the crops to survive until harvested. Many of the trace minerals essential to humans are not needed by plants, and these are not added to the soil, making the vegetables and fruit grown in that soil increasingly poor dietary sources of minerals.

White flour blues

That the essential nature of vitamins and minerals was discovered at all is due not only to clever chemical sleuth work but also to social changes in the early part of the twentieth century. Populations in search of work were migrating from rural areas to towns and cities, where the fresh country foods they had been accustomed to, like vegetables and eggs, were expensive and beyond their means. White flour was cheap, but the processing of flour to increase its shelf life stripped it of most of its vitamins and minerals. Certainly it filled hungry bellies, but it provided little nutrition.

Subsisting on a diet with a lot of white flour and sugar and little protein or good fats, the urban poor were sicker and died younger than their country cousins. Gradually, through careful experimentation—first on animals, and later on humans—it became clear that food contained not just one or two, but numerous different elements working together to keep us healthy. The realization that deteriorating health could be due to nutritional deficiencies changed medical thinking about the origins of disease. Up to that point only trauma, infection and frank extreme starvation were considered as causes of death and disease.

A little help in a stressful time

Alberta, June 2013. The flood of all floods. It starts in the northern part of the province. A slow-moving weather system is creeping east across central Canada, bringing exceptionally stormy weather. The rain seems endless. Within a few days a state of emergency is declared as rivers breach their banks and highways are flooded. By the middle of June, the threat of flooding is receding somewhat in the north, but the weatherman warns of more rain to come, this time centred on Calgary, Canada's fourth-largest city.

If there is such a thing as a perfect storm, this is it. A rapid thaw in the Rocky Mountains is sending meltwater tumbling into rivers below, while a massive rainstorm parks over Calgary, delivering days of unrelenting heavy downpours. After a brutally cold winter, the ground is still frozen and can't absorb the water. More than 100,000 people have to flee to higher ground, leaving behind most of their possessions. Rampaging floods and mudslides close highways; broken-hearted residents watch as cars are swept away and homes collapse.

As the floods subside, calls go out for help and the army is deployed to assist with the ensuing cleanup. Care packages are hastily assembled—underwear, toothbrushes and toothpaste, rubber boots and waders, brooms, buckets and mops. It will take a year, maybe more, for the city to rebuild and recover from the largest and most expensive natural disaster in Calgary's history to date.

Dr. Bonnie Kaplan, PhD, is a psychologist at the University of Calgary and a seasoned researcher who has spent many years studying the impact of vitamins and minerals on mental health. She is well aware of the increased demands for micronutrients under stressful conditions—several published studies have demonstrated that vitamin supplements can be helpful for people coping with similar unfortunate situations. Within a few weeks she assembles her team and they design a research project asking, Can the psychological stress caused by the aftermath of this terrifying disaster be eased with supplements?

Health Canada agrees to fast-track the regulatory approval process, and a large manufacturer provides the necessary supplements for the study.

Participants are assigned to take either vitamin D or a supplement containing high doses of the B vitamins. Another group gets a broad-spectrum combo of vitamins and minerals. For six weeks, these human guinea pigs are monitored for perceived stress, depression and anxiety.

When the results are analyzed, they show that those taking either the B-complex or the multivitamin and mineral supplement have experienced significantly less stress and anxiety compared with those only taking the single nutrient.[6] The strain of coping with the flood and its aftermath is just one extreme example of how stress makes greater demands on our nutritional resources.

Do healthy people benefit from additional vitamins and minerals?

While it may be agreed that the need for essential nutrients increases with age, stress and medication use, is there any reason to take supplements if you are neither old, a smoker or on medications? Will you notice any impact on brain function?

In a recent study, researchers gave fit, healthy young men a multivitamin and mineral preparation, one that contained levels of B vitamins ten to fifteen times the recommended daily allowances (RDAs) as well as vitamin C at eight to ten times the RDA. The RDAs are the officially recommended amounts of essential nutrients assumed to be sufficient to keep everyone of a particular age and sex healthy. After one month of treatment, testing revealed that compared to the men not taking the micronutrient cocktail, those in the treatment group were more upbeat and their mental processing was faster and more accurate, especially when put under pressure. They felt less stressed, had better memory, and they attacked exercise with increased physical vigour.[7] Remember that these are apparently fit, healthy young men not smoking or taking drugs, and eating a regular diet.

In the United States, a two-year Congress-mandated research project is currently underway to examine the evidence that supplements of vitamins and other essential nutrients can protect and enhance brain function and cognition in military personnel. Clearly, active military duty exposes soldiers to high stress levels, both physical and psychological, and any intervention that can help them deal with that stress would be welcome. But soldiers are not unique. As we will see in Chapter 6, anyone battling ongoing stress, either at work or in their private lives, can benefit from additional nutrients in the form of supplements.

The clinical experience of physicians and others who use vitamins and minerals in their practice and counsel patients on healthy eating patterns, as well as a growing body of research, suggests that healthy people of all ages may benefit from enhancing their diets with carefully selected supplements. However, it is important to remember that these are supplemental to and not instead of a good diet; supplements can never make up for poor eating habits. In particular, high intakes of vegetables and fruit confer special benefits.

Vegetables—The new essentials

Today we know that one of the main reasons for consuming a vegetable-rich diet is because it is high in more recently identified chemicals. We call these compounds phytochemicals, from *phytos*, the Greek for plant. Mounting evidence suggests that phytochemicals can protect us against an array of modern illnesses—from heart disease and stroke to diabetes and dementia.

Plants depend on sunlight to provide them with energy, which they capture through a process called photosynthesis that allows plants to convert carbon dioxide and water into carbohydrates and oxygen. During normal daylight hours, however, there will be periods when plants are exposed to more sunlight than they can handle. The resulting stress, called photo-oxidative stress, generates free radicals. The colour pigments of plants are antioxidants and work hand in hand with antioxidant vitamins and minerals to dissipate free radicals and protect cells against damage.

Like us, plants' DNA can be damaged by ultraviolet rays. But unlike us, they can't deal with excess sun by moving into the shade, covering up or slapping on sunblock. Plants therefore acclimatize themselves to excess sunshine by making their own natural sunscreens—the phytochemicals. A varied veggie-centric diet can provide a cornucopia of phytochemicals to combat oxidative stress and neuroinflammation. This is probably the mechanism whereby phytochemical-rich diets can enhance memory, learning and mental agility.[8]

Natural antibiotics

The soil plants grow in is teeming with potential pathogens—bacteria, viruses, fungi and moulds, even worms. Without the capacity to fend off these pests, a plant could never survive. So some of the phytochemicals they produce are antimicrobial and can repel, inhibit or kill these potentially problematic microorganisms. Some of these are as strong as any doctor-prescribed antibiotic. And since plants must be prepared to fight many different types of infections simultaneously, the phytochemicals they make are not just antibiotic, but also antifungal and antiviral too.

Many hospitals are experimenting with plant phytochemicals in the battle against hospital-acquired infections, especially bugs that have developed antibiotic resistance like methicillin-resistant *Staphylococcus aureus* (MRSA) or vancomycin-resistant *Enterococcus* (VRE). Oil of oregano, eucalyptus oil and tea tree oil, all popular home remedies for infection, colds and flu, can inhibit the growth of these superbugs.[9] The fact that plant-based antimicrobials are broad spectrum is a huge advantage when dealing with hospital-borne infections, since patients may be infected with more than one bug at the same time; they might have viral-bacterial or bacterial-fungal co-infections. And if you have a sore throat or a cough, it is sometimes difficult to know if the cause is viral or bacterial. Here again, plant-based antimicrobials like oil of oregano are a natural solution and should be staples in our medicine cabinets.

Forget five-a-day—It's ten-a-day

If you have bought into the idea that you should "aim for five" servings of vegetables and fruit every day, then it's important to know that this advice is no longer valid. In fact, it never was. Five a day (vegetables and fruit combined) is appropriate only for children between the ages of four and eight. The current consensus is that adults gain the most benefit from ten servings a day. A twelve-year study from the United Kingdom suggests that five servings a day or fewer had no impact on "all-cause mortality"—that is, the risk of dying for any medical reason.

People eating seven servings a day reduced their risk of premature death from heart disease, cancer or any degenerative disease by 42 per cent. But even though this was a clear advantage, it was not optimal. Researchers observed that the death rate continued to decline with every additional serving up to ten portions a day.[10] "The clear message here is that the more fruit and vegetables you eat, the less likely you are to die at any age. My advice would be, however much you are eating now, eat more," said the study's lead author, Dr. Oyinlola Oyebode, then at University College London's department of epidemiology and public health.

The study also found that vegetables outperformed fruit—they were up to four times more protective. Unlike whole fruit, fruit juice did not seem to be protective, while canned fruit increased the risk of dying by 17 per cent. It seems that at some point the benefits of the phytochemicals in fruit juices or canned fruit is offset by the extra sugar they contain.

What is a serving size? It's a baseball-sized piece of fruit, half a cup of cooked, chopped, or frozen fruits or vegetables, or a whole cup of raw leafy greens. Remember if you buy frozen fruit to make sure there is no added sugar. If you are unsure about serving sizes, check out the many websites, including those of government agencies, that show the serving size for different fruits and vegetables, or see the appendix at the end of this book.

Not as daunting as it seems

If you are dismayed at the prospect of consuming ten servings of vegetables and fruit, day in and day out, you are not alone. Not long ago I was visiting some friends in Dublin and the subject of diet came up at breakfast. "It's impossible to eat ten servings of vegetables and fruit a day," grumbled my host. "No one could do it."

His wife stopped him short. "Wait a minute," she said. "Let's just think about what we ate yesterday. At breakfast we had fresh fruit salad—at least one cup, and that's two servings. I went out for lunch with my friend and had a salad and a grilled chicken breast. I think that is at least three more servings. I had an apple with some cheese as a mid-afternoon snack, and with dinner we had two vegetables. That's eight in total. With a bit more effort I think I could stretch that to ten. Maybe we could have a salad every evening before dinner, and perhaps some berries for dessert instead of your usual bowl of ice cream."

Still grumpy, her husband responded, "That's all very well for you. You ate out for lunch and could order what you liked. I made myself a grilled cheese sandwich. No vegetables there."

"Well, if you had looked in the fridge, you would have seen a cucumber and some tomatoes. Couldn't you have chopped some of those up and eaten them with your sandwich?" his wife asked.

"I suppose so," her husband replied, "but I just didn't think of doing it."

And here's the nub of the problem. For most of us—even those of us who really like them—vegetables have not been a priority. Indeed, modern diets seem to place the highest priority on starchy carbohydrates like pasta, bread, potatoes and rice—high-glycemic foods that as we have seen increase the risk of most of the chronic diseases of aging, as well as Alzheimer's disease.[11] But if we can shift our thinking and fill our plates first with vegetables or fruits, they begin to displace the less healthy high-glycemic foods we love so much.

Chapter 14 includes a list of foods, mainly plants, that have been shown to be most protective for our brains. These form the basis for the MIND diet, which researchers have shown can protect against memory loss.[12]

It's hard to change overnight

While ten-a-day should become everyone's new mantra, don't expect to change overnight. At the back of this book you will find a fruit and vegetable diary that you can keep from time to time to see how you are doing. It's a good reality check and helps to get a baseline—find out how many servings a day your current diet provides and then, week by week, try to improve on that number. Remind yourself that for every daily increase over five the health benefits climb.

In Chapter 14 you will find some suggestions that will help you increase your daily intake of fruits and vegetables. And it need not mean banishment to the kitchen for a lifetime of peeling, chopping and shredding! Remember, it's a gradual process where you try each week to do a bit better than you did the week before. Eventually you will have achieved the ten a day you are aiming for. Typically I find that when someone achieves that magic ten a day, they wonder how they ever ate any differently.

Developing universal dietary guidelines

Following World War One, a new organization, the League of Nations, came into being. Its mandate was simple—to ensure that war never broke out again. Part of that effort was to make certain people were healthy and as well fed as possible. What type of diet would maintain health for most people at the lowest cost?

Various health committees were set up and conferences held involving leading experts in nutrition from around the world. Diets in Japan, the United States and South America were compared for their nutritional content. As the Great Depression set in, getting enough food for everyone was difficult, and the committee's deliberations took on a special urgency. Their 1935 report laid the groundwork for the development of eating guidelines in Canada and elsewhere.[13]

By 1937, the Technical Committee of the League of Nations was categorizing foods according to whether they were highly protective, less protective or non-protective. Protective foods included milk, cheese, butter and eggs, liver, fatty fish like herrings and salmon, green vegetables, salads and raw fruit. Cod liver oil was also in the highly protective group, since by that time the use of cod liver oil to prevent rickets and other bone disorders related to vitamin D deficiency was firmly established.

Less protective food included meat and root vegetables like potatoes and turnips, as well as legumes like dried peas and lentils, and cereals like bread and rice. Interestingly enough, there was no distinction between wholewheat and white bread—both were included in the less protective grouping. Sugar, jam and honey were considered non-protective, being high in calories while at the same time adding little nutrition. The committee also recommended 1 g of protein per kilogram of body weight, with substantially increased amounts for growing children and pregnant women.

Today the recommendation for protein intake is 0.8 of a gram per kilogram of body weight, decreasing with age until by seventy years of age it's 0.66 of a gram per kilogram of body weight.[14] But current research using more refined and accurate testing suggests that these recommendations for protein are too low. And far from decreasing with age, protein requirements actually increase.[15] Current research is also reaffirming the importance of the foods originally listed eighty years ago as highly protective. Apart from eggs and milk, these are foods that are not widely consumed by the general public. Fatty fish, green vegetables, raw fruit, eggs and milk do, however, form the foundation of the classic Mediterranean diet.

All in all, we seem to have made very little progress in defining healthy diets and educating the public in the last eighty years, or in weaning them off empty calories and on to foods that feed both body and brain. Our current diets are, unfortunately, heavily focused on the high-calorie, low-nutrient foods in the less protective and non-protective food groups identified by the League of Nations all those years ago.

No happy ending

I wish I could report that the case of the professor whose brain had stopped working had a happy ending. But it didn't. When she came to see me, she had taken a short leave of absence from her job and intended to use the time to try to get well—to de-stress, rest and recover. She knew she wasn't eating properly and wanted to learn how to improve that. She had a personal trainer and was trying to exercise regularly. A friend had suggested she might also benefit from vitamin supplements, which is why she had come to see me.

At that first visit she paid as close attention as she could to what I had to say. But in truth, she found it hard to follow. After all, what we were discussing was complex. I was explaining as clearly as I could the interplay of the many different nutrients needed for her brain to focus and concentrate, but I was exhausting her. She yawned frequently— a sure sign that her brain was working double-time trying to make sense of what I was saying, and using up more oxygen in the process. After a few visits she stopped coming to see me. From her friend I heard she gave up taking supplements, as well as regular exercise. Eventually she was forced to retire, finishing her university career prematurely.

It didn't need to happen. As you read through the remaining chapters of this book, you will see how important it is to be proactive about feeding the brain and will learn about optimal eating for all stages of life that will enhance learning, increase stress resilience and protect memory well into old age.

PART 2

When the Brain Stalls

CHAPTER 5

Alzheimer's and Dementia: Our Greatest Fears

The object of life is not to be on the side of the majority, but to escape finding oneself in the ranks of the insane.

Sometimes attributed to
ROMAN EMPEROR MARCUS AURELIUS

Thanks largely to modern medicine, we are currently enjoying record lifespans. But along with longer lives comes the increased burden of chronic disease: each passing year increases our risk of diabetes, heart disease, stroke, eye diseases, arthritis and osteoporosis. We call these diseases non-communicable or chronic degenerative diseases. Unlike the infectious diseases that caused the majority of deaths in earlier centuries, these conditions are not contagious. They don't get better on their own, and there are no antidotes.

Modern medical know-how can help us manage degenerative diseases. We can take drugs to control high blood sugar, cholesterol or blood pressure, the early warning signs of diabetes or heart disease. We can replace faulty heart valves and free ourselves from excruciating joint pain by replacing hips or knees. If kidneys stop working, we can be hooked up to a dialysis machine that will do their job or, if that fails, have a kidney transplant.

But one degenerative disease, dementia, has no medical fixes. Not at present, anyway. Despite the billions of dollars spent on drug development, all new medications have so far been spectacular failures, and drug companies are getting discouraged about further investment. Our best hope for now is prevention, and as we will see in Chapter 13, research consistently demonstrates that this is entirely possible.

However, prevention requires us to seriously rethink our lifestyles and, in particular, the way we eat.

Our greatest fear

According to polls, the prospect of getting Alzheimer's, the most common form of dementia, frightens us almost as much as cancer, and even more than a heart attack or a stroke. Perhaps this is because so many of us have witnessed in family and friends the devastating effects of this disease. First identified as a major and growing public health concern forty years ago, dementia is a relentlessly progressive disease. Dementia has been called "the long goodbye" because patients can live anywhere from five to twenty years after diagnosis.

First described in 1906, Alzheimer's disease is named after its discoverer, the German psychiatrist and neurophysiologist Alois Alzheimer (1864–1915). He examined the brains of patients who had died with severe memory problems, personality changes and impaired reasoning. Under the microscope, he saw fewer neurons and synapses than expected, and shortened or truncated dendrites and axons. Many cells were dead or dying. Scattered between the neurons were plaques—clumps of protein called beta amyloid—and twisted strands of tau protein. These plaques and tangles are characteristic features of Alzheimer's disease.

Plaques and tangles

Beta amyloid starts life innocently enough. It is found throughout the body and in the brains of all healthy individuals. At low levels it is not harmful. In fact, it is essential for normal brain function. Beta amyloid is needed to reinforce synapses. It assists in the growth and survival of nerve cells. It acts as an antioxidant, protecting neurons and glial cells from free radical damage. It supports the maturing of stem cells into neurons and plays an active role in damage repair.[1]

However, high levels of beta amyloid can aggregate into toxic clumps. These bind strongly to neurons, setting in motion a process that erodes synapses and eventually leads to the death of neurons. This good-guy, bad-guy role for beta amyloid may explain why drugs aimed at suppressing its production have not so far been helpful in the fight against Alzheimer's disease.

Tau protein has a normal function too, stabilizing microtubules, the hollow tubes of protein that give structure to cells. Microtubules form the tracks along which mitochondria travel within cells to provide energy where needed. They form the spindle along which chromosomes migrate when cells are dividing. They also form a vital transport system for the passage of nutrients into cells and the removal of waste products out of cells.

In the healthy brain, microtubules exist in nicely ordered parallel strands, similar to railway tracks. Like the wooden ties that keep railway tracks parallel, tau proteins help keep the strands parallel and unkinked. But damaged tau proteins can't perform this essential function, and the microtubules eventually degenerate and collapse into tangles—the tau tangles. Finally, deprived of physical support, energy and nourishment, neurons can no longer survive.

It seems likely that both beta amyloid and tau proteins interact to cause the brain dysfunction we call Alzheimer's disease. Researchers tracked 120 healthy men and women in their seventies for two years. They measured the amount of beta amyloid in their brains using brain scans and checked the amount of tau proteins in their spinal fluid. Each of these proteins seemed to enhance the toxic effect of the other, and interactions between the two appeared to drive the development of Alzheimer's.[2]

Not an equal-opportunity disease

About 70 per cent of Alzheimer's patients are women. This may be because women live longer than men, and the chance of getting dementia increases with age. But the dramatic drop in estrogen women experience after menopause also seems to be a factor. Estrogen helps with the release of the neurotransmitter acetylcholine, also known as the brain's "memory manager." Whereas men continue to produce estrogen as they age, in women production falls rapidly after menopause—the very years of greatest vulnerability. The estrogen theory is strengthened by research showing that, after menopause, estrogen replacement therapy offers women some protection against Alzheimer's.[3]

Although generally a disease of old age, Alzheimer's can happen to people in their forties and fifties. Then it is called early-onset Alzheimer's. Dementia at this age can be particularly devastating. Patients are likely to be at the peak of their careers and earning potential. Many still have young families to care for or may themselves be primary caregivers for a parent with dementia. And since doctors are not generally on the lookout for dementia at this age, initial symptoms may be misdiagnosed as depression or stress, and a correct diagnosis may take years.

The many faces of dementia

Although Alzheimer's is by far the most common form of dementia, there are other equally serious forms. They all involve the premature death of brain cells and a progressive deterioration of cognition.

Vascular dementia. A rich network of blood vessels nourishes the brain. With every heartbeat, up to 25 per cent of circulating blood is shunted through this network. Clearly, any factor that interferes with blood flow will limit the access of nutrients, oxygen and energy to the brain.

Raised blood pressure or dysregulated cholesterol—signs of poor cardiovascular health—are major risk factors for vascular dementia. Similarly, type 2 diabetes and obesity, which are linked to inadequate diet and poor cardiovascular health, are also risk factors. Calcium deposits in the walls of blood vessels make the small convoluted blood vessels that ferry nutrients deep inside the brain narrower and less flexible and more likely to become blocked.[4] Vascular dementia is the second most common form of dementia.

Lewy body disease. This form of dementia is caused by clumps of an abnormal protein called alpha-synuclein that accumulates inside neurons, dendrites and axons. These accumulations are called Lewy bodies. Apart from general mental decline, symptoms include movement problems, such as a shuffling walk, severe stiffness or tremors. Lewy bodies are a hallmark of Parkinson's disease, and their development in the brain may precede diagnosis by a decade or more. At the moment, the mechanism by which Lewy bodies contribute to dementia is not clear.

One characteristic symptom of Lewy body disease is visual hallucinations—the patient sees objects, animals and people that are not there and believes they are real. The disease is more common in men than in women and can progress rapidly.

Frontotemporal dementia and Pick's disease. The frontal lobes, situated behind the forehead, are responsible for planning and organization, motor skills, language and judgment. The temporal lobes, located behind the ears, process sound and are responsible for hearing and comprehension. Damage to the temporal lobes is linked to hearing loss, reduced speech fluency and inability to recognize familiar faces.

In frontotemporal dementia, brain cells shrink and die. In contrast, in Pick's disease, brain cells become enlarged and filled with clumps of tau protein, called Pick's bodies. Unlike Alzheimer's disease, these conditions often begin with marked changes in behaviour and personality. Patients have poor impulse control and exhibit abnormal social and sexual behaviour. Although they can exist separately, these dementias frequently occur together.

Mild cognitive impairment (MCI). When a noticeable deterioration in cognitive function beyond the normal changes seen with aging occurs, it is called mild cognitive impairment. Here memory is clearly impaired, but other cognitive functions are not compromised and daily living is unaffected. MCI is thought to represent a transitional stage between normal cognition and the development of full-blown dementia. More than half of those diagnosed with MCI will progress to Alzheimer's disease within five years.[5]

Explaining the inexplicable

A major problem with dementia is that it is often accompanied by disruptive and inappropriate behaviour, making coping with patients very difficult for their caregivers.

Nancy's husband, John, was diagnosed with Pick's disease in his fifties. Always a popular guy with a quirky sense of humour, John loved to tell stories. A diehard people watcher, he quickly picked up on little idiosyncrasies of behaviour he saw around him, spinning his observations into amusing anecdotes to entertain anyone who would listen. And people loved to listen. "John, tell us about the time that . . ." was a common opening gambit in conversations when he and his friends got together. The stories were so funny no one tired of hearing them again and again.

One early sign that something was wrong was when the retelling of old stories became obsessive and unprompted by requests. At a frantic pace, John would launch into one of his old yarns, sometimes to perfect strangers. Not many minutes later he would start recounting the same tale. It was no use reminding him that everyone had heard that story moments before—he just plowed on. Gradually it became clear that something unsettling was happening. Finally, John was diagnosed with Pick's disease.

Unlike Alzheimer's patients, patients like John retain their ability to remember day-to-day events and find their way around. But repetitive behaviours and obsessions become a problem. Patients often become preoccupied with food, overeating excessively and gaining huge amounts of weight. They may need to eat certain things at certain times every single day. At one point John became hooked on a particular brand of mints with a hole in the middle. He would wander around stores looking for them but wouldn't buy any until he'd opened each tube to check the shape of the mints. Telling him to stop was pointless. His wife simply followed him around, watching him like a hawk. Before they left the shop she would pay for all the opened mint packets.

These shopping incidents were the least disruptive of John's public behavioural problems, but his family treated each episode with awe-inspiring calmness and humour. At first they tried to explain his behaviour to strangers. Later, his wife had cards printed that simply said, *My husband has frontotemporal dementia or Pick's disease.* These she would hand to people she felt had been upset or embarrassed by her husband. "I never apologize for his behaviour," she said. "He is who he is and will only get worse."

She chronicled John's long illness in a blog, hoping that her family's experience and the ways they found to cope with it might help others in similar situations. John died from sudden cardiac arrest seven years after his original diagnosis.

The birth and death of neurons

One puzzling fact about the pathology of dementia is that the extent of plaques and tangles or Lewy bodies doesn't seem to predict the degree of cognitive impairment: the brains of individuals with perfectly normal behaviour and mental faculties contain many of these abnormalities.[6] And some loss of neurons—about 10 per cent—is perfectly normal during aging. This cell loss is mainly confined to the hippocampus, a region that interacts with the cerebral cortex to control emotions and process memories. The good news is, however, that cells in the hippocampus are capable of continual renewal.

The speed of new cell generation appears to be related to the degree of stimulation the brain receives; animal experiments show that presenting the brain with new challenges prompts the birth of new neurons. Out of this observation has grown a whole industry of computer-based brain games designed to keep brains active in middle age, and presumably dodge the bullet of dementia. Younger adults, too, have been encouraged to use brain-training games to enhance memory and to help them learn faster and better.

But do they work? Are they worth substantial investments in time and money? In 2014 neuroscientists at Stanford University and the renowned Max Planck Institutes in Berlin reviewed all the scientific evidence available and concluded that there was no convincing evidence to support advertised claims. "We object to the claim that brain games offer consumers a scientifically grounded avenue to reduce or reverse cognitive decline when there is no compelling scientific evidence to date that they do," their consensus statement read.[7]

On the other hand, an environment enriched with many different types of intellectual, sensory and cultural stimulation will continually improve neural plasticity and help preserve memory with age.[8]

More education = Fewer signs and symptoms

The more education a person has, the lower his or her risk of Alzheimer's disease. Each additional year of education corresponds to an 11 per cent decrease in risk of developing dementia. This is not to say that highly educated people are immune to the disease—even Nobel laureates have developed dementia.

There are several reasons why more years spent in education might be linked to better brain health in later life. Extended periods of formal learning could lead to the creation of higher numbers of synapses and more efficient and well-connected neural pathways. More educated individuals might therefore have greater brain reserves and cope better with the challenges of deteriorating cognition.

Research has shown that higher levels of education do not necessarily protect against the plaques and tangles associated with dementia. But those with more education do show fewer outward signs and symptoms of the disease while alive, suggesting they were better able to compensate and lead more normal lives.[9]

Alzheimer's—Many years in the making?

In Colombia, scientists have examined the brains of a large extended family known to have a high incidence of a gene called presenilin-1. Family members who carry this gene begin to have memory problems in their mid-forties and develop full-blown dementia in their fifties. Researchers tested family members aged eighteen to twenty-six, none of whom had yet developed memory problems. Some of them carried the gene, while some did not.

The gene carriers had higher levels in their blood and spinal fluid of beta amyloid, the protein thought to be responsible for Alzheimer's disease. Their brains were different too, and contained significantly less grey matter than those of non-carriers. Gene carriers had greater activation in the hippocampus, suggesting that it was working extra hard just to function.[10]

These physical differences were present nearly two decades before symptoms of dementia appeared, suggesting that brain changes are silently progressing long before any outward evidence of dementia appears.

Cigarettes, excess weight and empty calories

The World Health Organization has estimated that 14 per cent of dementias are caused by smoking.[11] Smoking also increases the risk of other chronic diseases, including cancer, lung disease, heart disease and diabetes—the latter two adding to the risk of developing dementia. So rule number one for long-term brain health is to stop smoking. Better still, don't start in the first place.

Worldwide obesity is projected to surpass tobacco use as the most important modifiable risk factor for all chronic diseases, including dementia. Should we be surprised? Although its development is complex, one underlying reason for the dramatic rise in obesity is the quality of modern food. It doesn't nourish us the way it should, and brains inevitably suffer. A "prudent" pattern of eating based mainly on vegetables and fruit, fish, nuts, seeds and whole grains appears to protect against both weight gain and dementia.[12] In contrast, typical Western diets, high in sugary drinks, processed meats and refined starches, not only increase the risk of obesity but are directly implicated in declining mental health.

Diabetes type 3?

In Chapter 3 we saw how eating a high-sugar, high-starch diet—that is, one with a high glycemic load—can paradoxically starve the brain of glucose and lead to insulin resistance. Insulin resistance in turn limits the flow of glucose and other needed nutrients into brain cells. As expected, insulin resistance and its consequence, diabetes, have a negative impact on all brain functions, reducing focus and attention and impairing executive function, planning, learning and memory. It is also a major risk for Alzheimer's disease.

Many researchers now refer to Alzheimer's disease as diabetes type 3 or diabetes of the brain. Indeed, insulin resistance and diabetes may be the common thread linking the classic features of Alzheimer's disease: neuronal cell loss, impaired brain energy and the accumulation of beta amyloid and neurofibrillary tangles.[13]

What about alcohol?

While it is agreed that long-term heavy drinking damages the brain, the effect of moderate alcohol consumption on health is hotly debated. While most studies show that moderate alcohol consumption offers some protection against Alzheimer's, others have found no benefit. Certainly, the evidence for protection is not strong enough to suggest that non-drinkers begin consuming alcohol in an effort to avoid the disease. Moderate alcohol intake is generally defined as two drinks a day for men and one for women.

Once Alzheimer's disease has been established, alcohol seems paradoxically to be more helpful. One study found that two to three units of alcohol a day slowed progression and lowered mortality in mild Alzheimer's disease.[14] So people in the early stages of Alzheimer's have no reason to forgo the pleasure of a cocktail or a glass of wine with dinner. An added problem in interpreting studies on alcohol consumption is that some researchers believe that the data itself is unreliable: when questioned about their drinking, research subjects may lowball their estimates, which could certainly influence research outcomes.

So, despite numerous studies, there is still no consensus on the role of alcohol in brain health beyond the certainty that chronic excessive drinking is detrimental.

"Smart carbs" and brain health

One way to ensure you're eating a low glycemic load is to swap out starchy carbohydrates, the mainstay of Western-style diets, for lower-starch vegetables and fruit, sometimes called the "smart carbs." These provide the continuous supply of glucose the brain needs without triggering the excess insulin production that starves brain cells of glucose. Since such a diet is lower in calories, it can also help prevent obesity.

But as we have seen, vegetables and fruit have benefits beyond their glucose content or calorie count. The phytochemicals they contain have powerful protective effects on the brain. Normal brain activity results in the release of free radicals, which can damage brain cells. Experts have linked excess free radicals to many illnesses, including cancer, diabetes and heart disease.

In later chapters we will explore how a phytochemical-rich diet can protect against the added burden of free radicals caused by stress, over-work or brain injury.

Dirty brain disease?

Remember how glial cells, the non-neuronal cells of the brain that out-number neurons by ten to one, were originally considered only minor players in brain function? It turns out that they are crucial in preventing the buildup of abnormal proteins and other cellular debris in the brain that occurs in dementia.

Throughout the body there is a drainage system—the lymphatic sys-tem—which is responsible for cleansing tissues of toxic waste produced by normal day-to-day metabolism, infection and wear-and-tear. Just as the blood supply circulates nutrients and oxygen, the lymph system also transports nutrients around the body, especially fats and proteins, as well as immune cells that fight infection and remove the remnants of dead and dying cells. Unlike the blood supply, which has the heart as a pump to keep blood circulating, the lymphatic system depends on the regular contraction of muscles to move lymph around, meaning regular physical exercise is essential.

Until recently the lymph system was not believed to extend into the brain, and how the brain self-cleansed was a bit of a mystery. But recent work confirms that the brain possesses its own lymph-like net-work, now dubbed the "glymphatic system" since it is managed by glial cells. Researchers have discovered that specialized glial cells—astro-glial cells—form channels along blood vessels entering the brain. This glymphatic system moves cerebrospinal fluid, the clear liquid sur-rounding the brain and spinal cord, deep into the brain, bringing with it immune cells, glucose and other nutrients, and flushing out dead cells and waste products like beta amyloid. The glymphatic system in turn is connected to the lymphatic system of the body, from where waste can be eliminated. The healthy brain appears to be able to self-cleanse in a more organized way and on a much larger scale than was previously understood.[15]

The glymphatic system works only while we sleep. Dr. Maiken Nedergaard, MD, of the University of Rochester Medical Center, a scientist at the forefront of glymphatic research, puts it this way: "The brain only has limited energy at its disposal and it appears that it must choose between two different functional states—awake and aware or asleep and cleaning up. You can think of it like having a house party. You can either entertain the guests or clean up the house, but you can't really do both at the same time."

Genes and dementia

Having a first-degree relative with Alzheimer's disease increases your risk of getting the disease by about 30 per cent. If this figure seems alarming, it's important to understand that this is your *relative* risk of acquiring Alzheimer's disease—in other words, how much more likely you are to get the disease compared to the general population. The relative risk of getting a disease is what usually gets quoted in media reports and university press releases, often because it makes a story seem more sensational.

But relative risk doesn't tell the whole story. To determine your personal risk you need to know the absolute risk of getting a disease, or how common a condition is in the first place. In the case of Alzheimer's disease, we know that eleven in every hundred individuals sixty-five years and older will develop the disease—that's an 11 per cent absolute risk. Having a parent or sibling with the disease increases your risk by 30 per cent of 11, or 3.3 percentage points. This gives you a 14.3 per cent absolute risk—not quite such a scary increase over the rest of the population.

Cholesterol and the brain

So much emphasis has been placed on links between elevated blood cholesterol and heart disease in recent years that we may have lost sight of the fact that cholesterol is an essential fat and needed for total body health. We use cholesterol to build cell membranes and to make estrogen, testosterone and adrenal hormones. It is the raw material the body converts into vitamin D when exposed to sunshine. The brain contains about 20 per cent of total body cholesterol, about 70 per cent of which is in the myelin sheaths of the axons of neurons, where it plays an important structural role. Cholesterol in the brain influences synaptic plasticity, learning and memory.

Because cholesterol is a large molecule—too large to cross the blood-brain barrier—the cholesterol that circulates in blood cannot access the brain, and the brain makes its own. Cholesterol is made almost exclusively by the glial cells, although a small amount is made by neurons. The manufacture of brain cholesterol, its metabolism and its excretion are all highly regulated, and upsetting this regulation can seriously affect brain health. Neurological diseases such as Niemann-Pick disease, Huntington's disease, Parkinson's and Alzheimer's disease have been linked to defects in cholesterol metabolism in the brain.[16] Drugs called statins (such as Crestor and Lipitor) that suppress the body's ability to make cholesterol are small enough molecules to cross the blood-brain barrier. Potentially, they could interfere with the brain's ability to produce necessary cholesterol.

Most medications carry a risk of side effects, but if the benefits outweigh the risks, they are usually continued. In the case of the statin drugs used to reduce cholesterol, there have been reports of brain-related side effects such as memory loss, forgetfulness and confusion.[17] The idea that statin drugs can negatively affect brain health is controversial, and some studies even suggest that these drugs may protect against Alzheimer's disease. However, other drugs that lower cholesterol have also been shown to negatively affect memory.[18]

What seems clear is that we don't have enough research yet to be sure that interfering with the regulation of cholesterol in the brain is safe for everyone.

Genes, cholesterol and Alzheimer's disease

Located on one of our chromosomes—chromosome 19—is a gene called apolipoprotein E (ApoE). It provides instructions for making a protein needed to transport cholesterol and remove amyloid deposits from the brain. This gene has three forms: ApoE2, ApoE3 and ApoE4.

About 20 per cent of the population are born with the ApoE4 version. This is the least efficient at clearing amyloid deposits and is known to increase the risk of Alzheimer's disease. Half the population have the ApoE3 variant, which doesn't pose a risk, while the least common form, ApoE2, is superefficient, and prevents beta amyloid accumulation. Those fortunate enough to have ApoE2 seem protected against Alzheimer's.[19]

Because we inherit an ApoE gene from each parent, we might have one, two or no copies of ApoE4. Not surprisingly, having two copies of ApoE4 further increases the risk of Alzheimer's disease. However, genes are not destiny. Most people who get Alzheimer's disease are not ApoE4 carriers, and many people with one or even two copies of the ApoE4 gene never get Alzheimer's. This is why genetic testing is rarely recommended. It's not really that informative.

Are supplements necessary?

While supplements cannot compensate for poor eating habits, government data from all developed countries, including Canada and the United States, show that the diets of many adults and children regularly fall short of recommended intakes of key micronutrients. The older we get, the more likely we are to suffer from deficiencies, especially of those vitamins and minerals critical for brain function, like vitamin C, magnesium and B vitamins. Supplements can then make up for shortfalls. So far, the strongest associations between supplement use and dementia prevention have been found for omega-3 fats, the B vitamins and antioxidants.

As we have seen, omega-3 fats play numerous roles in general health. In the brain, they serve as receptors for neurotransmitters and hormones, and enhance the ability of glial cells to remove amyloid plaques.[20]

In Okinawa, Japan, home to some of the world's healthiest older individuals, fish intake is high. Studies of elderly Okinawans show that the higher their blood level of omega-3 fats, the better their mental functioning.[21] So even in this fish-eating population, more seems to be better.

Unfortunately, present-day fish stocks cannot be guaranteed free of brain-damaging mercury or other pollutants, so converting to a high fish-based diet might not be the most helpful move for long-term brain health. A safer bet may be a daily supplement of fish oil, since most commercial products are screened and guaranteed pollutant free. In mild cognitive decline, the benefit of omega-3 fats has been shown to be enhanced with a high intake of B vitamins—further proof that no single nutrient works alone.[22] Fish oil supplements may also somewhat offset the detrimental effect of heavy alcohol consumption.[23]

Is it dementia or B-vitamin deficiency?

Of all the vitamins and minerals that work together, none cooperate more closely than the B vitamins. As in a family where one child is singled out for more attention than its siblings, favouring one B vitamin over the others can create disharmony. For example, two members of the B family—folic acid and B12—work closely together. The relationship between these two has been severely distorted by the modern practice of adding folic acid to our food. Both Canada and the United States currently fortify food with folic acid, and many countries are debating whether to follow suit.

Folic acid is the synthetic version of the folate found in green leafy vegetables. We add it to food to protect women from having a baby with spina bifida. But in order to use folic acid, the body must convert it to its active form, methyltetrahydrofolate. This conversion needs B12. An imbalance of these two B vitamins—too much folic acid and insufficient B12—is a growing concern and has been linked to birth defects in babies and memory problems in the elderly.[24] In Canada, 4 per cent of adults have blood levels of B12 below 148 pmol/L, which is considered deficient. However, even blood levels much higher than this are linked to deteriorating brain health and age-related cognitive decline.[25] In Japan and Europe, the lower limit for serum B12 is between 500 and 550 pg/mL.

If left untreated, B12 deficiency can cause irreversible damage to the brain and nervous system. Indeed, the symptoms of prolonged B12 deficiency are easily confused with vascular dementia. B12 interacts with the ApoE4 gene, and ApoE4 carriers with low B12 may be at increased risk of cognitive problems. For example, they have been shown to have increased difficulties with facial recognition.[26] In patients already diagnosed with mild cognitive impairment, high-potency B-vitamin supplementation can slow the rate of progression to full-blown Alzheimer's disease.[27]

Antioxidants and risk of Alzheimer's disease

The brain is a target for attack by free radicals—rogue molecules that cause damage to cell membranes and DNA. Free radical damage disrupts normal cell functioning and eventually triggers the death of neurons. The control of this attack depends on high circulating blood levels of antioxidant nutrients, including vitamins A, C and E and the minerals manganese, selenium and zinc.

The body also counteracts free radical damage by producing its own antioxidants (endogenous antioxidants), such as superoxide dismutase (SOD), coenzyme Q10 (CoQ10) and glutathione. Although we can make these molecules ourselves, their synthesis will depend on availability of other nutrients in our diets. For instance, the manufacture of SOD depends on the availability of copper, while glutathione requires vitamins C and E, B vitamins and the minerals selenium, magnesium and zinc as co-factors. Deficiencies of any of these essential nutrients therefore limit the amount of antioxidants we make.

The phytochemicals found in colourful fruits and vegetables have been shown to block the production of free radicals, preventing damage to mitochondria and shielding neurons from toxicity. In later chapters, you will read more about how high blood levels of these antioxidants protect the brain, and how they work together to shield delicate brain tissue from damage.

Putting the D in dementia

Receptors for vitamin D can be found throughout the brain and on neurons and glial cells. This fact alone suggests that vitamin D is integral to normal brain function and that vitamin D deficiency is likely to have a detrimental effect on brain health. Vitamin D activates and deactivates enzymes involved in neurotransmitter synthesis, preserving healthy levels of dopamine and serotonin in the brain. It protects neurons from toxins and reduces inflammation.[28]

One study found that those with deficient (less than 50 nmol/L 25-hydroxy D) or severely deficient (less than 25 nmol/L) vitamin D levels circulating in their blood had more than double the risk of getting Alzheimer's disease.[29] Patients followed for nine years in the Framingham Heart Study had reduced hippocampal volume and poorer mental functioning if their vitamin D levels were low.[30]

Recent findings suggest that the activated form of vitamin D—1,25 dihydroxyvitamin D—is needed for the uptake and absorption of the insoluble beta amyloid plaques by glial cells, so that they can be flushed out of the brain through the glymphatic system. Insufficient vitamin D handicaps these cells and allows the plaques to accumulate. Omega-3 fats also play a critical role in promoting the destruction and removal of beta amyloid, and it has been suggested that the combination of low levels of vitamin D and omega-3 fats could trigger the onset of Alzheimer's disease.[31]

Since we commonly see inadequate intakes of both these nutrients in older adults, this suggestion should ring alarm bells.

Why we can't ignore the oil light

If nutritional inadequacy is a major risk factor for Alzheimer's disease, can taking supplements or changing diet help once dementia is established? Perhaps, but maybe only in the early stages. In mild cognitive impairment, for example, progression to full-blown Alzheimer's can be halted with supplemental B vitamins. And correcting a B12 deficiency can reverse the signs and symptoms of B12 dementia, which mimics vascular dementia.[32]

However, if a B12 deficiency continues for long enough, permanent neurological damage can occur that is likely to be irreversible, regardless of supplementation. Think of it this way: when your car's oil light goes on, you know your oil is getting low. If there is a gas station nearby and you replace the oil quickly, no harm is done. But if you ignore the red light and continue driving, the engine will eventually seize up and the car will grind to a halt. No amount of oil can help at this point—the damage is irreversible. A careful car owner regularly checks the oil and tops it up before it gets too low.

Similarly, if we want to avert cognitive decline, diet and supplements will be most effective when used for prevention rather than treatment. In Chapter 13 we will discuss regimes that can help if the oil light does go on and memory becomes a concern. But because the seeds of Alzheimer's may be sown long before symptoms appear, it's never too soon to start making healthier dietary choices. Don't wait for the red light to come on.

CHAPTER 6

This Is Your Brain on Stress

If you ask what is the single most important key to longevity, I would have to say it is avoiding worry, stress, and tension. And if you didn't ask me, I'd still have to say it.

GEORGE BURNS,
How to Live to Be 100—Or More

New clients frequently mention stress as a health concern. Perhaps they are dealing with a recent diagnosis of cancer and wonder if the considerable stress they were under prior to diagnosis had contributed in any way. Or maybe a condition like Crohn's disease or lupus that has been in remission has recently returned. Why now, they ask? Could stress have anything to do with it?

Some level of stress is normal and perfectly healthy. It keeps us alert and helps us perform well under pressure. But too much stress certainly affects health and can both trigger new health problems and make pre-existing conditions worse.[1] A particularly strong link exists between stress and brain health. At any age, from childhood into old age, exposure to extreme or prolonged stress can reduce neural plasticity, interfering with the formation and strengthening of synapses that are essential for learning and memory.[2]

Excessive stress is a major player in the development of mood disorders like anxiety and depression. And increasingly, chronic stress is seen as a trigger for the development of dementia. It could be the stress of a prolonged illness or major surgery, or years of family or work-related stress. Any or all can result in the development of the initial symptoms of dementia—mild cognitive impairment—or spur the progression of MCI to full-blown Alzheimer's disease.[3]

A new syndrome is born

The term "stress" was first used in a medical context in the 1930s by Hungarian Canadian Dr. Hans Selye, MD (1907–82). Before then it was simply an engineering term—the stress on a bridge is the load it can carry before it is damaged. As a medical student in Montreal, Selye noticed that all patients who were ill had one thing in common regardless of what was wrong with them: they looked anxious, pale and fatigued. They seemed defeated by their condition and no longer able to cope. Selye wondered why wildly different illnesses result in these same common endpoints. Could this "syndrome of being sick" be defined in precise scientific terms?

Selye's research showed that there was indeed a predictable sequence of biochemical and pathological events that occurred when the body had excessive demands placed on it. There were hormonal adjustments, largely driven by the adrenal glands. Over time, he found, these changes led to the development of many different health problems: stomach ulcers, high blood pressure, atherosclerosis, arthritis and even allergic reactions.

In the short term, hormones released by the adrenal glands are protective after trauma or injury. They work in our favour—or rather, they are helpful if we are attempting to escape life-threatening situations. Release of stress hormones heightens our awareness, making us hyper-vigilant to clues from our environment—clues that could be vital for our survival. Stress hormones dampen down inflammation and numb us to pain. Blood flow is directed away from non-critical functions like digestion and towards muscles and the brain, allowing both tissues to increase their uptake of glucose and oxygen and work harder.

All of which is fine if we are attempting to rescue a drowning child or flee from a marauding animal looking for its next meal. Under those circumstances we need to be able to think on our feet and summon up sudden bursts of energy—maybe even superhuman strength. But what if the stress persists and the release of stress hormones is prolonged? Then, Selye showed, widespread and often irreversible damage occurs. And not just to one organ, but throughout the body.

His seminal paper on the topic, "A Syndrome Produced by Diverse Nocuous Agents," was published in the journal *Nature* in 1936.

Not one stress, but many

When we think about stress we usually mean psychological stress. Bereavement, a messy divorce, troubled teenage children—all are given full credit as burdens on our health. But Selye showed that stress came in many different guises. Although it frequently *was* psychological, it could also be physical: exposure to excessive heat or cold, heavy manual labour or extreme forms of exercise. Stress might be medical, resulting from surgery, chronic pain, lingering infection or prolonged drug treatment. Or we could be stressed by our environment; pollution, excessive heat and noise all triggered the stress response.

Stress could even be joyful, like falling in love, travelling or winning the lottery. As Selye wrote in his 1974 book *Stress without Distress*, "The mother who is told her only son has died in battle suffers a terrible mental shock; if years later it turns out that the news was false and the son unexpectedly walks into the room alive and well, she experiences extreme joy. The specific results of the two events, sorrow and joy, are completely different, yet their stressor effect—the non-specific demand to adjust herself to an entirely new situation—may be the same."

And Selye pointed out that different types of stress are cumulative. Both small and large stressors combine to defeat us; like the stress on a bridge, it is the total load that is important. Which is why, when we are under extreme stress, it is often the straw that breaks the camel's back—the trivial frustration that makes us finally explode. All types of stress ultimately cause similar health effects. Overworked, the adrenal glands weaken and eventually stop functioning because they have exceeded their ability to cope.

The hormones of life

Perched like little caps on top of each kidney, the adrenal glands are where the main stress hormones originate. Anatomically the glands consist of two distinct regions—the outer layer or cortex, and an inner region called the medulla. Each region secretes its own distinct stress hormones.

The adrenal cortex makes steroids like aldosterone, which controls blood pressure and the body's salt and water balance. It also produces cortisol, a hormone familiar to most of us. Cortisol regulates our blood sugar and controls the conversion of fats, proteins and carbohydrates to energy. It dampens down inflammation and suppresses certain aspects of immunity. Synthetic versions of cortisol like prednisone and cortisone are used to treat an overactive immune system in inflammatory conditions like rheumatoid arthritis.

In a healthy person, cortisol levels vary over the course of the day. They are generally highest in the morning shortly after we wake. Then, as the day progresses, they drop to reach their lowest levels overnight. After a sudden stress like an accident or an argument, cortisol briefly rises, regardless of the time of day. When the stress is resolved, cortisol should normalize. However, if stress is ongoing, cortisol levels may remain high throughout the day. High cortisol levels can lead to chronically elevated blood pressure and blood sugar, rapid weight gain, anxiety and depression. Too little cortisol throughout the day, on the other hand, can cause fatigue and weight loss.

Cortisol and the brain

In the brain, surges of cortisol direct blood away from the prefrontal cortex, responsible for problem solving and impulse and emotional control, and reroute it towards the hindbrain—the so-called reptilian brain. Located in the brain stem, the reptilian brain controls the instinctive reactions needed for survival. This primitive part of the brain has no memory but influences our heart rate, body temperature and breathing.

As well as the reptilian brain, early mammals developed a more sophisticated brain system, the limbic brain. The limbic system is known as the emotional centre of the brain because it allows an animal to remember the events or situations that produce pleasant or unpleasant sensations and respond accordingly. The limbic system is not one discrete region but three—the hippocampus, amygdala and hypothalamus—which together work to manage our response to threats.

Although we often use alcohol to unwind at the end of the day and coffee to wake up in the morning, excess alcohol and caffeine both increase cortisol. Since cortisol levels need to be low to enable us to sleep, consuming too much of either before bed is a bad idea. On the other hand, if you feel like a wet rag in the morning until you have had several cups of strong coffee, perhaps your cortisol is too low in the morning and normal biorhythms are out of sync.

A sustained high blood cortisol level can cause damage throughout the brain. In the prefrontal cortex, it weakens synapses and reduces neuronal firing.[4] Over time, the hippocampus shrinks in volume. The birth of new neurons ceases and working memory is impaired. The risk of severe memory loss and dementia increases.[5]

The other adrenal hormones

The other region of the adrenal glands—the medulla—secretes two hormones, adrenaline and noradrenaline (also confusingly known as epinephrine and norepinephrine). Noradrenaline is also secreted from nerve endings throughout the body, and by neurons in the brain. It is our "fight or flight" hormone. Adrenaline and noradrenaline prepare the body for the vigorous response needed to fight a threatening situation, or to get out of the way of trouble double-quick. They are released after a strong emotional response, such as fear of an attacker or of almost being run over by a car. Adrenaline and noradrenaline will be released while waiting for a job interview or a dental appointment.

The release of adrenaline causes a sudden burst of physical and mental energy, sometimes called an adrenaline rush. This will increase heart rate and blood pressure. We sweat, our lungs expand to take in more oxygen, our eyes open wide and our pupils dilate. We may experience palpitations or a rapid heartbeat. Whereas the hormones secreted by the adrenal cortex are essential for survival—we die without them—those secreted by the medulla are not.

Which doesn't mean that they are not extremely important: when adrenaline and noradrenaline are dysregulated we feel the effects very strongly.

Burnout, nutrition and the brain

Our brains are vulnerable to burnout if we subject them to work overload. Modern imaging techniques that follow the uptake of nutrients into the brain show that the harder we work our brain, the more nourishment it uses. So it shouldn't surprise us that permanent damage can occur when the nutrients the brain needs for daily repair and maintenance are regularly undersupplied. Even occasional shortfalls can cause the brain to stall, affecting our performance at work and our enjoyment of leisure and family time.

Deficiencies of vitamins, minerals, essential fats and amino acids needed for moment-to-moment brain function are widespread: even in those who consider themselves healthy eaters, these nutrients are frequently undersupplied. And although the food we eat is of fundamental importance, hard-working brains benefit from additional nutrients in the form of supplements to ensure optimal function and maintain brain health. As we saw in Chapter 4, when healthy, fit young men were given a multivitamin with B vitamins that were ten to fifteen times higher than the current RDAs and then subjected to stress, their mental processing was faster and more accurate. Even their exercise endurance improved.

Clearly, the addition of such supplements would give them an edge at work and at play.

Conditionally essential nutrients

Under stress, certain elements of diet not classically thought of as essential can become a factor. We call these nutrients "conditionally essential" because their biosynthesis is limited in certain situations. Vitamin D is a good example of a conditionally essential nutrient. Strictly speaking it is not a true vitamin since we can make it ourselves. But since we need ultraviolet rays to make it, vitamin D becomes essential when there is a lack of sunshine.

Coenzyme Q10 (CoQ10), a major antioxidant, is another example of a conditionally essential nutrient. It is needed for mitochondrial function. We need to take supplements of CoQ10 if we take cholesterol-lowering statin drugs, because statins block not only the synthesis of cholesterol but also of CoQ10.

As the basic building block or precursor for adrenaline and noradrenaline, the amino acid tyrosine is also conditionally essential. We can get quite a lot in our diets when we eat protein. We can also manufacture it from another amino acid, phenylalanine, which is similarly present in protein-rich meals. However, tyrosine becomes essential when we are under stress. Then, no matter how well we eat, our diet is unlikely to provide enough to meet all our needs.

Tyrosine is required to make many critical molecules essential for our metabolism, and it is not difficult to imagine dietary tyrosine supplies being overwhelmed by demand. We use it to make thyroxine, the thyroid hormone, and to make melanin, the pigment of skin and hair. It is the building block for CoQ10 and is also required to make the endorphins or enkephalins—the natural painkillers of the body. But one of tyrosine's most critical tasks is to make dopamine, a neurotransmitter that, as we have seen in previous chapters, plays a crucial role in controlling brain function.

The stress of chronic pain

We sometimes forget how stressful chronic pain is, and how draining it can be. I remember one client who came to see me, whom I'll call Michael. When he was quite young, Michael was diagnosed with a serious form of arthritis, and he had lived with pain most of his adult life. Now in his fifties, he needed crutches to walk.

Over the course of a year he began to benefit from a comprehensive regime of vitamins and minerals. In particular, low vitamin D was corrected and his magnesium intake optimized, since deficiencies of both these nutrients are linked to musculoskeletal pain. He generally ate well and avoided junk and heavily processed food, but we tweaked his diet further, eliminating added sugars and substantially cutting back on starchy carbohydrates. In due course, he was able to give up his crutches and needed only a cane to walk.

Convinced stress had a major impact on his pain, he decided to leave his demanding job and take early retirement. When I asked him how he intended to spend his retirement years, he smiled and admitted that his secret passion—a passion he had not been free to indulge much while he was working full-time—was writing poetry. Now he intended to focus on it seriously. My immediate response was that he might benefit from tyrosine supplements. Dopamine is a key neurotransmitter involved in creativity, and tyrosine supplements have been shown to ramp up creative thinking.[6] Dopamine influences the creative drive by allowing a flood of sensory stimuli into the brain. In artistic individuals, this can lead to an awareness of unusual patterns—of words, images and sounds—and an enhanced ability to come up with novel ideas.[7]

Since pain is only one of many stressors that can deplete tyrosine, it made sense that supplementing with it to boost dopamine might help Michael with his writing. And so he started taking 2,000 mg of L-tyrosine every morning when he woke, waiting thirty minutes before eating. This was to allow the tyrosine to enter his brain without competition from other amino acids. A few days later I received an email from him that said everything I needed to know in one sentence: "Wow—it's like I've found the on-switch for my brain!"

The dopamine brain drain

What is the link between tyrosine, dopamine and stress, and why do individuals experiencing any form of stress benefit from tyrosine supplements? To answer that question, we need to understand one very basic metabolic pathway. You see, dopamine is rapidly depleted when we are under stress, because it is used to make the stress hormones noradrenaline and adrenaline.

Dopamine → noradrenaline → adrenaline

After an adrenaline surge, we can top up depleted dopamine if we have enough circulating tyrosine. But if we don't, we will certainly feel the consequences. Lack of dopamine will leave us feeling fatigued, depressed and lacking in motivation. Concentration and focus will suffer. And of course, without enough dopamine we will not be able to make additional noradrenaline or adrenaline should we need to.

The fact that dopamine gets used up to make stress hormones is mostly overlooked by mainstream medicine. But I believe it is the real reason stress makes us feel so bad. Lack of dopamine explains most of the symptoms associated with extreme or chronic stress. It is also the reason that tyrosine supplements are so useful—they can replenish dopamine stores even as they are being drained by the adrenal glands.[8]

Who benefits from tyrosine supplements?

Anyone experiencing a traumatic life event, like a divorce or bereavement, will find tyrosine supplements helpful. It doesn't numb the pain like medications do, but it does increase the ability to cope. Supplementing with tyrosine also decreases stress-related increases in blood pressure and has been shown to improve brain function in situations wherever there are high demands.

Multiple studies have shown that tyrosine can counteract the reduction in working memory and information processing that occurs in healthy individuals whenever they are confronting a demanding situation. It might be brain overload from work, a job loss or even extreme weather conditions.[9] Since dopamine is needed for word recall, public speakers will find that it improves fluency: anyone facing a nerve-wracking presentation or social situation will find tyrosine particularly helpful.

Athletes can take it to increase stamina, focus and concentration.[10] I frequently recommend it to golfers, who take it before a match and often find that it improves their game. A pianist I introduced to tyrosine supplements was able to abandon medication for performance anxiety, and felt that his playing also improved. Getting older is stressful to some people, and as a matter of course I suggest it to those in their seventies and beyond. Tyrosine can help by dampening down the increased stress reactivity that often accompanies aging.

Post-traumatic stress disorder

Although it has been around for a long time, post-traumatic stress disorder (PTSD) was formally recognized as a medical condition only in 1980. Exposure to unusually harsh forms of stress such as torture or witnessing violent or life-threatening acts can all lead to PTSD, as can sustained physical or mental abuse. While some people are able to put a scary or shocking event behind them after a while, others seem to get locked into the fight-or-flight response and continue to feel stressed or frightened months, years or even decades afterwards.

Active military duty exposes soldiers to heavy physical and psychological demands, and they are at high risk of developing PTSD. Tyrosine supplements have been shown not only to increase mental and physical performance in military personnel, but also to help prevent PTSD.[11] In fact, many of the studies showing the benefits of tyrosine supplements were originally carried out in the armed forces. In the United States, a two-year Congress-mandated research project is currently underway to examine the evidence that supplements of vitamins and other essential nutrients can enhance brain function in military personnel and perhaps protect against PTSD. However, anyone battling ongoing stress, either at work or in their private lives, can benefit from similar regimes.

I prefer to introduce tyrosine supplements when no other changes in supplements or diet are taking place. This way clients can see for themselves whether they benefit. First, I ensure that other co-factors needed to make dopamine are in place. I make sure the client has been taking a good-quality multivitamin for at least a month. I also need them to be taking omega-3 fats, as well as extra vitamin C and magnesium.

The water-soluble B vitamins seem especially important. As we have seen, under stress we benefit from additional B vitamins at levels much higher than currently recommended. While some multivitamins contain only current RDA levels of B vitamins, others contain higher levels. Look for one that contains a minimum of 25 mg of B6.

Vitamin C and stress

As we saw in Chapter 4, vitamin C is a powerful antioxidant, protecting the brain from free radical damage. Most animals make their own vitamin C, from glucose. Unfortunately, one of the genes needed to do this mutated in primates, so we cannot synthesize our own vitamin C and must depend on our diets to provide enough. Evolutionary biologists speculate that animals without the ability to make vitamin C survived only because they lived in an environment abundant in vitamin-C-rich foods. Manufacturing vitamin C consumes a lot of energy—energy that would have been in short supply for early humans. So possessing this mutation would have provided primates with extra energy to survive and flourish in an energy-poor nutritional environment. But today we have no need for extra energy; modern diets typically contain too many calories. And we certainly don't eat enough vegetables and fruits, the foods rich in vitamin C.

In 2009, a study of university students in Toronto between the ages of twenty and twenty-nine found that one in seven had vitamin C blood levels normally associated with scurvy, while a further one-third had suboptimal levels. Despite their youth, those with low blood levels of vitamin C had elevated blood pressure, body weight and waist circumferences, as well as signs of inflammation in their blood normally associated with an increased risk of heart disease.[12]

High vitamin C stores are found in both the adrenal cortex and the medulla, which may explain why vitamin C supplements alter blood levels of both cortisol and adrenaline. Vitamin C is needed to make neurotransmitters like dopamine and serotonin, and to generate noradrenaline and adrenaline. We might guess therefore that under stress we would need extra vitamin C, and we would be right. As you can see from the table below, animals capable of making their own vitamin C not only make a lot more vitamin C per kilogram of body weight than we think appropriate for human health; they also respond to stress by dramatically increasing their output.

Let's assume an average person weighs seventy kilograms; his recommended daily allowance of vitamin C is 75–90 mg. But if that individual were a goat of similar weight, we can deduce from the table that he would be making approximately 2.3 g of vitamin C daily. That is, provided the goat was completely unstressed, perhaps just nibbling grass in a field all day. If that same goat were stressed or became ill, its daily output of vitamin C would increase to an astonishing 13.3 g. This ability to ratchet up vitamin C production under stressful conditions is common to all animals that can make vitamin C, from mice to elephants. Surely this shows how central vitamin C is to the biological response to stress?

Species	Lowest daily requirement (mg/kg/day)	Highest requirement, stressed or ill (mg/kg/day)
Goat	33	190
Rat	39	199
Mouse	34	275
Rabbit	9	226
Dog	5	40
Humans (RDA)	0.9	None given

Source: Adapted from M. Levine, "New Concepts in the Biology and Biochemistry of Ascorbic Acid," *New England Journal of Medicine* 314, 14 (1986): 892–902.

To date, no research has systematically tried to understand our needs as human animals for vitamin C when we are ill or under stress. Guinea pigs are another mammal that cannot manufacture vitamin C. Initially they were the laboratory animals of choice for research, because like us they depend on diet to provide enough vitamin C. But we don't use these animals much anymore because, unable to adapt to stress by ramping up vitamin C production, they die too easily under the inevitable stress of experimental conditions and ruin our experiments.

Even guinea pigs kept as pets are very stress susceptible and display all the symptoms we associate with stress. They may become irritable and aggressive, or depressed and less active. They can also develop diarrhea, hair loss or skin problems—the early signs of scurvy. The stress might be a family dog that barks a lot or constant loud music. Or it could be fluctuating temperatures; guinea pigs must be kept away from drafts or they will die.

If we were guinea pigs

In the 1970s, researcher Man-Li Yew was working at the University of Texas at Austin. Aware that there was much argument about the human requirement for vitamin C and whether our needs increased under stress, he turned his attention to guinea pigs. Did their needs increase when they were stressed or ill? If so, he could be pretty sure that humans too would have increased vitamin C needs when they were stressed.

He took groups of healthy young guinea pigs, put them on diets containing varying amounts of vitamin C and then subjected them to the stress of surgery. The animals felt no pain because they were anesthetized. But although anesthesia blocks pain signals from reaching the brain, it doesn't stop the hormonal and metabolic changes that usually accompany trauma or injury.

Before and after the surgery their growth rate was monitored (these animals were the guinea pig equivalent of teenagers). Then Yew observed how rapidly they were able to heal and how quickly they recovered from anesthesia. To prevent scurvy, the animals needed only 1.5 milligrams per kilogram of body weight each day (mg/kg/day). This is slightly more than the RDA for humans at 0.9 mg/kg/day. But for ideal growth they needed 16 mg/kg/day, and for optimal recovery from anesthesia and surgery they needed much more—50 mg/kg/day.

If tissue requirements for vitamin C were similar in humans, these numbers suggest a child or teenager weighing 30 kg (66 lb.) would need approximately 1,500 mg a day for normal growth and development. And an adult weighing 70 kg (154 lb.) would need at least 3,500 mg a day to recover from surgery. As Yew noted, studies in guinea pigs only allow us to speculate about human needs under stress, but, he insisted, "The burden of proof must now shift to the medical scientists who are really concerned about the health and physical condition of young people to show that considerations that apply to young guinea pigs do not also apply to young people."[13]

A recent study of cardiac patients involved giving them either a placebo or 2 g of vitamin C intravenously just before surgery and oral doses of 1 g daily for the first four days afterwards. Patients given extra vitamin C had shorter hospital stays and fewer surgical complications.[14] Extreme exercisers who took 1,500 mg of vitamin C after a marathon had strikingly lower cortisol levels than are typically seen. Similar effects have been seen when exercise stress was combined with heat stress: those given extra vitamin C had lower cortisol levels after exercise.[15]

Perhaps it is high time to re-evaluate human vitamin C needs, and this time focus on stress and healing.

Magnesium and stress

One nutritional need that is clearly not being met by modern diets is magnesium, a mineral required to convert tyrosine to dopamine, noradrenaline and adrenaline. There is no argument that we are not getting enough—surveys in North America and around the world show most of us are not achieving daily recommended intakes. In the United States, less than half the population does so.[16] In Canada about 40 per cent of young adults consume too little, and this figure rises sharply with age; nearly 70 per cent of men and women seventy-one years and older fail to meet daily requirements.[17]

Magnesium is essential for our response to stress. Without sufficient magnesium we cannot manufacture neurotransmitters or use hormones. We need it for glucose metabolism and energy production. Magnesium keeps the digestive system working, heart rhythm steady and blood pressure under control. However, stress hormone release depletes magnesium by increasing its excretion in urine. So when we are magnesium deficient, stress becomes a double-whammy, compromising our ability to mount an appropriate stress response while also making that deficiency worse. In both animal and human studies, magnesium depletion has been shown to increase anxiety.[18]

I think there is a good biological reason that depletion of magnesium occurs under stressful conditions. Magnesium works in partnership with calcium to help muscles function. Muscles contract in the presence of calcium, and relax when there is an appropriate supply of magnesium. When muscle stores of magnesium are low, muscles can't relax and we feel tense. Our shoulders feel like they need a massage 24/7, we get leg cramps and back spasms, and irritating little muscle twitches show up in our eyelids or lips. We may get constipated or feel uncomfortably full hours after we have eaten even a small meal because the smooth muscles that control the passage of food through our digestive tracts can't relax properly.

On the other hand, when tissues are saturated with magnesium, we are not anxious and our bodies feel comfortable and relaxed. Epsom salts are magnesium sulphate, and anyone who enjoys an Epsom salts bath before bed will attest to their muscle-relaxing action. But relaxed muscles are hardly ideal for dealing with an emergency. The fight-or-flight response requires us to tense up, not relax. And to do this we need to offload magnesium—which may be why stress depletes it.

We will return to magnesium and explain how you can maintain good body stores later in the book.

Managing stress

Apart from reducing our intake of alcohol and coffee, which in moderation are both fine but in excess can increase cortisol levels, there are many proven ways to help us deal with stress.

Exercise is important for many reasons but is particularly valuable for stress management.[19] Regular exercise can reduce blood pressure, anger and hostility. However, extreme exercise can have negative effects. Overworking the body can result in the depletion of nutrients and physical injuries—damage to joints that may be difficult to rehabilitate. There is even some evidence that while moderate regular exercise protects against most chronic diseases, excessive exercise reduces healthy life expectancy.[20]

Massage therapy and maintaining strong, positive personal relationships have both been shown to reduce inappropriately high cortisol levels. And we can train ourselves to be less responsive to stress—to chill out—using cognitive behavioural training. Mindfulness-based stress reduction is a technique based on Buddhist traditions that is gaining in popularity. It has been shown to reduce cortisol and the symptoms of stress in a variety of mental and physical disorders. But healthy individuals under stress can benefit too.[21]

Seeking a preventative approach to health care, a new breed of doctors is emerging. Known as integrative physicians, they use both conventional medicine and a wide range of alternative or traditional medical approaches to promote health and healing. They focus on diet and nutritional repletion, but also exercise, acupuncture, yoga and tai chi, and manual therapies like chiropractic and massage to treat the whole person—mind, body and spirit. Integrative medicine is increasingly attractive to patients and is also finding a toehold in North American hospitals, universities and medical schools.

Stress management is central to the practice and philosophy of integrative medicine. One could say that the integrative physician is at last addressing the implications of Hans Selye's research.

CHAPTER 7

Brain Injuries:
Trauma and Stroke

Success is to be measured not so much by the position that one has reached in life as by the obstacles which he has overcome.

BOOKER T. WASHINGTON,
Up from Slavery

It is late afternoon and I'm sitting on the dock at a friend's cottage with several other guests. The day has been lazy, mostly spent swimming and reading. This evening we will catch up with each other's news, but for now we are silent, enjoying the serenity of our surroundings and relaxing in a way that city life precludes. In front of us the lake is a photographer's dream, its looking-glass surface perfectly reflecting the rocky shoreline and cloudless sky above. In the distance, joyful shrieks are heard as children jump off rocks and docks, enjoying a last swim before dinner.

This is a quintessential summer day in cottage country, northern Ontario, Canada. With our sun-soaked brains firmly set on idle, work and city life fades into the distance and a wordless communication with nature takes over. For a couple of days we can fantasize about living the simple life—the rustic cottage, the wood stove, the cooking and sharing of food—with a few city luxuries thrown in for good measure. As if reading our minds, our hostess appears on the dock carrying a tray of glasses, frosty from ice-cold wine.

Suddenly, several speedboats appear and begin criss-crossing the lake, churning the formerly calm water into sizable waves. Trailing behind them are large inflated inner tubes in which children of various ages ride. As each boat hits a wave a great shudder runs through it, and the tube that follows bounces wildly. The children cling on for dear life, screaming their heads off. Again and again each child's head is thrown backward and forward in a series of rapid, jerky movements.

"Sound like they're having fun," one of my companions on the dock comments, without looking up from her book. But as I watch their young heads jolt back and forth I cannot help but imagine the jelly-like brains of these young kids shifting back and forth, colliding repeatedly with their hard skulls. What damage is this doing? And if this joyride is regular weekend "fun," could any harm be cumulative?

Traumatic brain injuries

I might not have worried about the brains of the children at the lake had we not in recent years been forced to confront the damage done to the brains of professional sports players, especially those in hard-hitting contact sports like hockey and football.

For some years there had been whispers about possible long-term brain damage in professional football players. Off the field, many got themselves into hot water with the law, often for domestic violence. Initially this was attributed to the innately violent nature of the sport. Somehow the necessary hostility and aggression players were required to display on the field, or at the ice rink, spilled over into their private lives. Players were simply conditioned to have a lower threshold for anger and violence.

But many symptoms couldn't be explained away so easily. Some players were experiencing short-term memory loss. Some had developed movement disorders reminiscent of Parkinson's disease, or walked as if they were drunk. And among retired players there was clearly an increased risk of suicide.

Punch drunk

New Jersey pathologist Harrison Martland, MD (1883–1954), first observed brain damage from sport in professional boxers. His paper "Punch Drunk," published in 1928, begins, "For some time fight fans and promoters have recognized a peculiar condition occurring among prize fighters which, in ring parlance, they speak of as 'punch drunk.'

Fighters in whom the early symptoms are well recognized are said by the fans to be 'cuckoo,' 'goofy,' or 'slug nutty.'"[1] Examining deceased boxers' brains, Martland saw extensive neuronal cell death and neurological deterioration. He called this condition chronic traumatic encephalopathy, or CTE. Now we know that you don't have to receive repeated hard slugs to the head to develop CTE; mild blows or repeated shaking can do it too.

In 2008, Boston University School of Medicine established a brain bank to study the brains and spinal cords of eighty-five people who had experienced recurrent mild traumatic brain injuries during their lives. Of these eighty-five, sixty-four had been athletes, twenty-one had been military veterans (most of whom had also been athletes) and one had been a head banger, whose injuries were assumed to be self-inflicted. Not all the examined brains had the tell-tale signs characteristic of CTE, but in the sixty-eight individuals who did, the brain damage was extensive—localized in some brains but widespread in others—and ranged from accumulated neurofibrillary tangles to loss of axons in white matter.

The symptoms these individuals had experienced prior to death included headaches, loss of attention and concentration, depression, explosive rage and short-term memory loss. Those who had had the most aggressive personalities also had the most severe brain damage and were more likely to have been diagnosed with dementia at the end of their lives. In the thirty-four American football players included in the study, the longer they had played the game, the greater the brain damage.[2]

Is damage to kids' brains more severe?

When I was a child our parents thought little of it when we banged our heads, as inevitably we did. If we fell—off climbing frames, swings or monkey bars—we'd cry for a bit and maybe have a large egg-shaped bump on our heads the next day. But only an open wound was considered a serious enough injury to require a doctor. The idea of subtle injuries that could have long-term effects on our brains never entered our parents' heads. No one ever checked for changes in mood, or focus and concentration.

Today we know that head injuries in children that initially seem mild can result in long-lasting and even severe complications. A blow to the head may not cause loss of consciousness, but serious memory problems can develop later. Symptoms can be subtle at first—heightened anxiety, poor concentration, irritability or mild depression, and difficulty settling down to schoolwork. While most problems resolve spontaneously, they can become chronic.[3] Repeated impacts are more serious in young children than in adults. One study of football players found that they had poorer performance on neuropsychological testing as adults if they had started playing contact sports before the age of twelve.[4]

The myth persists that children are more resilient to brain injury than adults, so younger players are often allowed to return to playing sooner, sometimes the day after an injury. Before full recovery, however, less force is required to produce a second concussion, and symptoms are likely to be more severe and last longer.[5] Lack of symptoms immediately after an accident does not necessarily mean there is no damage; one study found that children who were initially symptom free did have neurological symptoms when examined two weeks later.[6]

Dr. Robert Cantu, MD, author of the book *Concussions and Our Kids*, thinks that the structural damage seen in the brains of adult athletes often begins at a young age. "All the research I've seen indicates that youth brain injury is a bigger thing than the same amount of brain trauma to an adult," he says. "Youths recover from brain injury, on average, more slowly than adults ... they can have quite profound changes in cognitive, behavioral and mood problems later in life from a brain injury early on."[7]

Strokes and the death of brain cells

A stroke is another form of brain damage, which occurs when the blood supply to part of the brain is interrupted or severely reduced. Brain tissue in the affected area is then deprived of nutrients and oxygen. Within minutes, brain cells begin to die. A stroke often results in paralysis, which may or may not be reversible.

There are two main types of stroke: ischemic strokes, where a clot forms that blocks a blood vessel, and hemorrhagic strokes. A hemorrhagic stroke occurs when an artery ruptures, allowing blood to spill into the surrounding tissues, causing compression. The rupture may be due to a malformed blood vessel, which could have been present from birth. Or it could be due to an aneurysm—a weak area in a blood vessel that bulges out under pressure and eventually bursts.

Like a stroke, but usually lasting only a few minutes, a transient ischemic attack (TIA) occurs when there is a brief interruption of blood flow to the brain. TIAs are often called mini-strokes. Most last only two to ten minutes, although some may last up to twenty-four hours. TIAs usually cause no permanent damage but can be a warning sign of an impending stroke: about a third of those who experience a TIA will go on to develop a stroke. Most strokes, however, are not preceded by a TIA.

The danger zone

After a stroke, two distinct regions of injury are seen on brain scans. At the hub or core of the injury, cells that are damaged beyond recovery die. Sandwiched between these dead cells and the healthy brain cells further away from the injury is a region known as the penumbra. Here cells have been stunned by the injury but are not irretrievably damaged. However, if blood flow to this region drops below a certain threshold these cells will die too, amplifying the original damage. In other words, a vicious cycle develops in which the initial injury leads to radiating death in cells not initially affected. Like a stone thrown into a still pond, where the ripples spread out from the initial centre of impact, progressive damage to healthy tissue follows.

Since the area of penumbral tissue that survives is closely linked to the degree of recovery from a stroke, the focus of emergency treatment is on salvaging these cells. To make sure they recover, blood flow needs to be restored to the penumbra as quickly as possible. A blood clot can be removed surgically, or drugs may be given that dissolve it—so-called clot-busting drugs. Since time is of the essence, these drugs must be administered within four and a half hours after a stroke. Treatment with aspirin, which is anti-inflammatory, and a blood thinner can also prevent new clots from forming.

Although they have different causes, strokes and traumatic brain injuries (TBIs) share some of the same biology. In TBIs an area of reduced oxygen and glucose metabolism develops around a central core of dead or dying cells. As with strokes, this can lead to the death of nearby healthy brain cells in the penumbra, and salvaging cells in this area is essential to prevent escalating damage.[8]

Are some TIAs brain cramps?

While some medical experts consider that TIAs and ischemic strokes are both caused by blood clots of differing degrees of severity, others believe that the vasospasm characteristic of TIAs and sometimes preceding a stroke is caused by cramping of the muscle layer within blood vessel walls.[9] This muscle layer, called vascular smooth muscle, contracts and relaxes to redistribute blood to areas where it is needed; the muscle contracts to supply areas that need more oxygen and relaxes in areas that need less.

As we saw in the last chapter, magnesium is needed for muscle cells to relax, and therefore sustained contraction, or spasm, suggests local tissue stores are inadequate. Leg cramps, back spasms, stomach cramps or esophageal spasms are all linked to low tissue magnesium. Cardiac arrhythmias and high blood pressure are also signs of magnesium deficiency—in fact, poor vascular health in general is linked to inadequate magnesium.[10]

The magnesium needs of the brain are high, and in a person with ample magnesium intake they are maintained at a higher level than found in blood.[11] A sudden drop in magnesium in the muscle layer of the blood vessels feeding the brain could possibly precipitate an ischemic stroke or TIA. This theory is supported by animal studies in which pre-feeding with magnesium can reduce the amount of damage that follows an experimentally induced stroke.[12]

The life and death of neurons

Cells die in two ways. In the first, necrosis, damaged cells simply burst apart. As they do so they release enzymes and other inflammatory molecules into the surrounding tissues. We generally know when cells are dying by necrosis because it generates inflammation, and that causes pain, swelling, redness and warmth at the site of an injury.

But there is another way cells die—by apoptosis. Apoptosis is a more regulated and systematic process by which the body eliminates cells that are unnecessary, unhealthy or simply aging. It is also called programmed cell death or cell suicide. Before dying by this method, cells carefully enclose their enzymes in membrane-wrapped parcels for disposal. There is no inflammation and we are unaware it is happening. Too little or too much apoptosis can be a problem. Too little, and cells that should be eliminated, like cancer cells, may persist. Conversely, unregulated apoptosis can inflict devastating tissue damage and is linked to the development of Parkinson's disease, Alzheimer's and other neurodegenerative disorders.

Magnesium may have a role to play in preventing inappropriate apoptosis after a stroke or other brain injury. Calcium drives apoptosis, pushing through channels (calcium channels) in the neuron's membrane and into the mitochondria. Once there, calcium triggers a cascade of events, and "death signals" that result in the demise of the neuron are released. Drugs called calcium channel blockers have been tried in patients with acute brain injuries either from trauma or bleeding. Theoretically they should work, but most studies have met with little success.

Magnesium is known as "nature's calcium channel blocker" and, at least in the laboratory, magnesium can interfere with rampant apoptosis, commuting a cell's death sentence. Some clinical trials have shown magnesium to be of some benefit after a stroke, even when administration is delayed for up to six hours.[13] However, the results of more recent, larger trials have been disappointing.

A fine balance

The reason that many clinical trials of magnesium for prevention of unnecessary apoptosis after a stroke or head injury have not panned out may relate to difficulties gauging the correct dose for individual patients. When magnesium is consumed in food or as supplements, the body has difficulty absorbing too much. Excessive magnesium over-relaxes the smooth muscle of the colon, causing diarrhea, which eliminates any excess. This is nature's way of protecting us from overabundant intakes of magnesium.

But in emergency situations—after a head injury or stroke—oral supplements are not considered practical, and all clinical trials so far have administered various doses of magnesium intravenously. Intravenous administration bypasses the protective role of the gastrointestinal tract, so too much magnesium may get into the blood. This can be dangerous—remember that magnesium relaxes muscles and that the heart is a muscle. Erratic heart rhythms and even cardiac arrest can result from too much magnesium in the blood.[14] If excess magnesium gets into the injured brain, it may even induce the very cell death it was meant to prevent.[15]

Compared to our hunter-gatherer forebears, we live in a calcium-rich, magnesium-poor nutritional environment and ingest a dramatically different and non-physiological ratio of calcium to magnesium. That this change increases the risk of stroke is clear from the fact that countries with the highest ratios of calcium to magnesium (high calcium/low magnesium) in soil and water have the highest incidences of cardiovascular disease and stroke.[16] As we saw in Chapter 6, stress depletes magnesium but doesn't appear to affect calcium. So high-stress lives may further magnify the calcium-magnesium imbalance caused by modern diets.

A study summarizing all the available evidence on the relationship between magnesium intake and risk of stroke found that the more magnesium people consumed from diet and supplements, the lower their risk of a stroke. For every 100 mg increase in magnesium intake there was an 8 per cent decrease in strokes, and this was consistent across all the studies examined.[17] Magnesium is one of several nutrients important for brain health for which dietary intake in North America is undisputedly inadequate.[18]

Magnesium can also protect against experimental traumatic brain damage in animals, speeding recovery; conversely, magnesium deficiency makes injuries worse.[19] So, in those recovering from a brain injury, whether from a stroke or TBI, oral magnesium supplements may help to prevent cells in the penumbra from dying. Intravenous administration of magnesium may also help, but it is fraught with pitfalls, since the dosage does not usually take into account the calcium status of the patient.

The best outcomes are likely to be seen in those whose magnesium intake was good to begin with, which would not only reduce the initial likelihood of a stroke but speed recovery from brain injuries whatever their origin.

Calcium in all the wrong places

While calcium can be highly toxic, especially in the context of brain injuries, at the same time it is also critically important for health. Not only is it the major component of bones and teeth, where it gives structural support, but electrically changed calcium—calcium ions—are involved in every aspect of how cells function, controlling processes as essential and diverse as fertility, tissue repair, learning and memory.[20] As we have already seen, a high intake of calcium can be damaging when magnesium intake is low. If there is a shortage of vitamin K, calcium may also become a problem.[21]

Vitamin K is a fat-soluble vitamin needed to manufacture vital proteins made by the liver called Gla proteins. Because these proteins are required for normal blood clotting, vitamin K deficiency causes excessive bleeding.[22] This is why in most countries one of the first things a newborn baby is given is a shot of vitamin K, just in case they are deficient. Otherwise babies are vulnerable to a bleeding disorder called hemorrhagic disease of the newborn. This condition can trigger spontaneous bleeding, and if it occurs in the brain, can cause extensive brain damage.

So far, seventeen Gla proteins have been discovered. One of these, osteocalcin, works with vitamin D to regulate the deposit of calcium into bones and teeth and is important for preventing osteoporosis and dental cavities.[23] Another Gla protein called matrix Gla protein prevents abnormal deposits of calcium that can occur in soft tissues like breasts, kidneys, heart valves and blood vessel walls.[24] Calcium deposits are undesirable because they interfere with vital processes in tissues where they occur. In arteries they cause hardening and narrowing, limiting the delivery of oxygen- and nutrient-rich blood to where it is needed.

Arterial calcification is a risk for stroke and dementia, and research is underway to see if vitamin K supplements might play a role in preventing this.[25] The recommended daily allowance of vitamin K is 90–120 mg/

day. However, higher levels may be needed for Gla proteins to be fully activated and prevent calcification.[26] While studies are very preliminary, doses of 500 mg and more of vitamin K2 can improve vitamin K status and slow the progression of coronary artery calcification.[27] There is no upper limit for vitamin K, and vitamin K supplements are very safe. Studies of vitamin K and osteoporosis have used daily intakes up to 45 mg (45,000 mg) without adverse effect.[28]

Be prepared!

Following a stroke, a TIA or a TBI, broad-based nutritional support is vital for recovery.[29] The nutritional needs of the brain—high to begin with—increase due to the metabolic stress of the injury. The injury triggers a cascade of molecular events that produce high levels of damaging free radicals, increasing the need for antioxidants.

Phytochemicals—the colour pigments of plants—are some of the most potent antioxidants available. They are plentiful in a diet rich in fruits, vegetables, herbs and spices, and can combat neuroinflammation and protect neurons against injury from free radicals.[30] As we have previously seen, eating ten servings of vegetables and fruit a day offers optimal health protection. Adults achieving this daily level of intake are best prepared for recovery from brain damage. Higher dietary and blood levels of vitamin C have been shown to reduce the risk of stroke.[31] All the antioxidants act synergistically, so a combination of vitamins, minerals and phytochemicals is likely to be most effective.

All nutrients essential for brain health have a protective effect when examined in clinical studies. Supplementing with the B vitamins, for example, is linked to a reduced risk of stroke and cerebral hemorrhage.[32] In Philadelphia, researchers examined the current diets of patients attending an outpatient traumatic brain injury clinic. Their daily intake of fourteen key micronutrients considered important for brain health was assessed, as well as their physical, emotional and cognitive health following the injury. Most patients failed to consume RDAs for many of the micronutrients. The more micronutrient insufficiencies a patient suffered from, the poorer their test results.[33]

Leg cramps and toxic drugs

I first got to know Margery when she was in her early seventies. Although retired from teaching, she led a busy life. Each morning she could be found at one of her many volunteer jobs: at the local hospital, acting as docent at the museum or delivering meals on wheels to the housebound. Every afternoon her grandchildren visited after school. She supervised their homework while they waited for their parents to come home from work.

She came to see me professionally at the suggestion of her doctor. Her energy was decreasing and her spirits were low. Her blood pressure was steadily increasing. She was curious if I thought a change of diet or vitamin supplements could control her creeping blood pressure and help her regain some of her former joie de vivre.

Certainly her diet could be improved. Although she didn't eat much junk food, she cooked a lot of the deep-fried, starchy and sweet foods beloved in her native Ukraine. Given her age, she was not eating nearly enough protein to maintain muscle mass and strength, and her fruit and vegetable intake was well shy of the ten servings needed for the best long-term health.

Discussing her health history, I discovered that Margery suffered badly from constipation, and had done as long as she could remember. In middle age she had developed debilitating leg cramps, mainly at night, for which she had been prescribed quinine. Quinine is an old-fashioned antimalarial drug that gives tonic water its distinctive bitter flavour. It is now no longer used for leg cramps because of its eye toxicity. Although present in only minute amounts—one-tenth the dose used to prevent malaria—even the quinine in tonic water can have toxic effects.[34]

A happy ending

I suggested that quinine was at best masking Margery's symptoms, without getting at the root cause of her leg cramps. Since magnesium deficiency is linked to both leg cramps and constipation, I suspected that lack of magnesium could be responsible for both problems. Her doctor felt she should stop the quinine, and Margery agreed to very gradually increase her intake of magnesium to "bowel tolerance," as outlined in Chapter 15 of this book.

She took to the dietary reforms I suggested like a duck to water and also adopted the supplement regime I recommended: a multivitamin with high levels of B vitamins, some extra vitamins C and E, 4,000 IU of vitamin D and a daily teaspoon of fish oil. As her constipation resolved, her blood pressure started to come down. Her energy improved and her bubbly personality re-emerged. Although she still got an occasional cramp, they had diminished greatly in frequency and severity. Margery seemed to have high needs for magnesium, which in her case I suspected could be genetic. Overnight, blood levels of magnesium fall and are lowest between 4:00 and 8:00 a.m.[35] I suggested to Margery that she should watch for signs of early-morning low magnesium blood levels, which might make her feel dizzy, nauseous or faint.

One morning her husband came down to breakfast to find her slumped in a chair and unresponsive. She was rushed to hospital where they suspected she might have had a stroke. The usual emergency protocols for stroke were immediately put into action—medications to thin her blood and break up any blood clots that might have formed and caused a blockage. That evening I called the hospital to find out how she was and I was put through to her directly. "I'm fine," she told me. "Apparently there is no physical or neurological damage." But she complained about the hospital food, which she said was unhealthy and unappealing.

I promised to visit her next day with a selection of foods I thought she might enjoy. However, I had no time to shop before I got a call to say she had been discharged. Since then she has not had a similar event. Now in her mid-nineties, she has no physical or cognitive signs she ever had a stroke. I like to think that she was helped by consuming all the nutrients that have been shown to speed recovery and prevent that ripple effect of brain cell death in the penumbra.

I also believe that had she continued to treat her leg cramps with quinine rather than address an obvious magnesium deficiency, her recovery might not have been so rapid and complete.

Nutritional support for recovery from stroke or brain trauma

While the best chance of a full recovery seems to be in those who are fit and well prepared nutritionally—exercising regularly, eating wholesome diets and achieving healthy levels of vitamins and minerals—anyone can take steps to speed their return to full health after a brain injury.

As support for basic maintenance and repair, the diet and supplement regime outlined in Part 5 should be implemented as soon as possible. Make sure that the multivitamin included contains higher levels of B vitamins (25–50 mg of each B vitamin). Here are some additional tips that may help to optimize recovery after brain damage.

Get a good night's sleep. Sleep is usually less efficient after either a stroke or a TBI—it may take longer to fall asleep, and frequent waking during the night is common. The protein clumps associated with Alzheimer's disease are also found in the brains of people who have had a head injury, and their accumulation may explain the increased risk of Alzheimer's disease after strokes and TBIs.[36] As we saw in Chapter 5, sleep is essential to allow the glymphatic system to efficiently clear these protein clumps from the brain.

Sleep is also essential for the production of melatonin. In experimental models of both stroke and traumatic brain injury, melatonin has been shown to be neuroprotective, reducing inflammation and protecting both grey and white matter.[37] If sleep becomes a problem, follow the nutritional protocol for insomnia described in Chapter 15.

Increase antioxidant supplements. As we have seen, antioxidants can thwart the escalation of damage and inflammation that can occur days or even months after a brain injury. Doubling the dose of vitamin C suggested in the basic supplement regime can be helpful. C-reactive protein (CRP) is a blood marker of inflammation, and high CRP levels that persist after a concussion are linked to worse outcomes.[38] Vitamin C supplements can lower CRP.[39]

Alpha lipoic acid is a powerful antioxidant that has additional advantages in that it can help to regenerate other antioxidants like vitamins C and E. It also recycles coenzyme Q10 and glutathione—two powerful antioxidants we make ourselves. While we do make lipoic acid in small amounts, most of it comes from diet. Rich sources are red meat, especially organ meats like kidney, heart and liver. Vegetable sources include spinach and broccoli. At least in animal models, lipoic acid supplements have been shown to speed recovery after a TBI or stroke.

Two forms of lipoic acid are found in commercial supplements: the R form and the S form. The R form is the form found in food and the one we synthesize ourselves, and some studies suggest it is the more effective of the two. Most supplements contain either the R form alone or a 50/50 mixture of the R and S forms. I recommend 300 mg of the R form twice a day. Take it between meals, because food appears to reduce absorption.

Ensure ample protein intake. Of all the macronutrients, don't neglect protein. The demand for protein increases after TBIs and strokes. As we saw in Chapter 3, we cannot store protein, so within one to three days of not meeting protein needs we start to cannibalize muscle tissue to provide the necessary amino acids to make critical hormones and neurotransmitters.

Protein needs may vary from 1.2 to 1.5 grams per kilogram of body weight per day depending on the type of injury and the degree of inflammation present.[40] These needs are easily overlooked, especially as patients recuperating from a stroke may have difficulty eating. Nausea is common after a TBI and appetite may evaporate. As we have previously seen, the daily allowance of protein should not all be consumed at one meal, but divided up throughout the day.

Whey protein is a practical source not only of the amino acids needed for brain repair, but also of lactoferrin, an effective anti-inflammatory and anti-infective protein found only in milk.[41] Available as a powder, whey protein can be incorporated into soups and smoothies.

Cut out added sugar and reduce starchy carbohydrates. Sugars and rapidly absorbed starchy carbohydrates like bread, crackers and other refined grain products cause blood sugar and insulin to spike after consumption. Good blood sugar control profoundly affects heart health and extends life expectancy after stroke.[42] Maintaining steady blood levels of blood glucose also improves outcomes in TBIs.[43] Hemoglobin A1c (HbA1c) is a blood test that estimates glucose control over a three-month period and is therefore a useful measure of how well an individual is controlling blood glucose and insulin levels. Ideally HbA1c should be less than 5.7.

Increase vegetable and fruit intake (and don't forget the fat). Anyone eating the ten daily servings of vegetables and fruit every day *before* a stroke or TBI will be in better shape to make a full recovery. But after a brain injury, the phytochemicals in vegetables and fruit become even more significant. All adults need to achieve their "daily ten." Children should consume an age-appropriate number of servings (see below). The era of fat-free salad dressings was a disaster as far as phytochemical nutrition was concerned, dramatically reducing their absorption. So don't forget to eat each of the daily ten with a little fat.

Recommended number of vegetable and fruit servings per day

2-3 years	4-8 years	9-13 years	14-18 years		19 years +
Boys and girls	Boys and girls	Boys and girls	Boys	Girls	Adults (both sexes)
4	5	6	7	8	10

Source: Health Canada, "How Many Food Guide Servings of Vegetables and Fruit Do I Need?," http://www.hc-sc.gc.ca/fn-an/food-guide-aliment/choose-choix/fruit/need-besoin-eng.php.

Smoothies are an excellent approach to increasing phytochemical intake post-stroke or TBI. They can be consumed through a straw over several hours if appetite is low or eating is physically difficult. If possible, include three to four servings of vegetables and/or fruit and one scoop of whey protein powder per serving. But be careful: it's easy to make a smoothie with a high glycemic load. Stick to the less sweet fruits—apples, pears, blueberries, et cetera—and above-ground vegetables. Fat can be added using avocado, nut butters or coconut oil.

One Food Guide serving is a medium fruit; half a cup of chopped, frozen or canned vegetables; or one cup of leafy salad greens. The Health Canada website gives examples of serving sizes of individual vegetables and fruits (http://www.hc-sc.gc.ca/fn-an/food-guide-aliment/choose -choix/fruit/serving-portion-eng.php).

PART 3

Back to the Beginning

CHAPTER 8

Brain under Construction: Diet and Pregnancy

"It's brain," I said; "pure brain! What do you do to get like that, Jeeves? I believe you must eat a lot of fish, or something. Do you eat a lot of fish, Jeeves?"

"No, sir."

"Oh, well, then, it's just a gift, I take it; and if you aren't born that way there's no use worrying."

P.G. WODEHOUSE,
My Man Jeeves

Opening my email one morning, I see a message I have been expecting—a birth announcement. Attached are photographs of a beautiful baby girl, the first child for a couple in their early thirties. The baby weighed in at a healthy seven pounds, eight ounces, neither too big nor too small. And although labour was long and exhausting, the delivery was uneventful.

At four weeks old, the baby is feeding well and mercifully giving her parents reasonable stretches of sleep at night. She seems to know when it's nighttime. Instead of waking every three hours to feed as she does during the day, during the night she will sleep at least six hours. Although the baby books say she is too young to smile—if you think your baby is smiling, they say, she's just puckering up to pass gas—her parents and doting grandparents think otherwise. "We look right at her and smile, and she smiles right back," they insist.

I don't doubt it. I know how well fed this baby has been from the moment she was conceived, and she is showing all the signs of the neurological maturity I have come to expect from babies carefully nourished in utero. For several years now I have worked with her parents. Although they have always eaten well, at my suggestion they gradually fine-tuned their diets to reflect the growing research literature on healthy eating. Their lifestyles are healthy too. They exercise regularly, don't smoke and drink only modest amounts of alcohol. Where possible they try to eat organic produce and limit their exposure to environmental toxins.

They planned carefully for this pregnancy: both were taking a vitamin and mineral supplement regime designed to support fertility and optimize the neurological development in any offspring they might conceive. In my dream world, every baby would start life under similar circumstances.

Brain health begins before we are born

For decades now it has been clear that, nutritionally speaking, the first few years of life are absolutely critical. Good maternal diet can set the stage for a healthy and uncomplicated pregnancy, and better health in infancy and throughout the entire lifespan of that baby. Incontrovertible evidence shows that as adults, the risk of acquiring chronic diseases like diabetes, heart disease or dementia begins before we are born.[1] And it's not just future disease risk that's at stake, but also intellectual development.[2]

Most of our lifetime's supply of neurons—an estimated 80 to 100 billion—are produced in an exuberant burst of proliferation during pregnancy, particularly in the last few months. Farmers know that during periods of rapid growth plants need precise and careful feeding to produce the healthiest and most abundant crop. Why should the nurturing of 100 billion neurons deserve any less attention? Since a baby's brain is rapidly developing during pregnancy, it makes intuitive good sense to support that growth with the best possible food. Food and the vital nutrients it contains are, after all, the construction materials for the developing brain.

The Barker hypothesis

In 1990 British researcher David Barker (1938–2013) first proposed that poor nutrition during pregnancy affected the lifelong health of a baby. His research suggested that babies born full term but unexpectedly small for gestational age—five pounds or less—were more likely to develop health problems as they grew older.[3] Being born small for gestational age meant that the baby's physical growth had somehow been constrained during pregnancy. While this had several possible explanations, the principal cause of growth restriction in an otherwise normal pregnancy is inadequate nutrition.

Adults who had been small as babies were shown to have increased rates of heart disease and strokes, as well as insulin resistance and type 2 diabetes. They were at risk for several types of cancer. Surprisingly, these tiny newborns were also more likely than normal-weight babies to become obese adults. Initially Barker's ideas were met with skepticism, but over the next decade his hypothesis was confirmed. From countries like India with high levels of poverty to comparatively wealthy countries like Finland or Great Britain, the research was conclusive: being born small for gestational age almost always reflected a mother's diet before and during pregnancy, and had profound and lasting effects on her baby's health.[4]

Is the brain protected when nutrition is in short supply?

Barker believed that the brain was a privileged organ: if there had been any shortage of nutrition during pregnancy, the baby's brain would get the lion's share at the expense of other organs. While to a certain extent this is true—the brain does appear to fare better than other organs when nutrition is in short supply—it would be surprising if undernutrition during pregnancy did not somehow affect brain development. As we have already seen, the brain has higher, much higher, nutritional requirements than any other organs.

When IQ testing is used to measure brain development, some studies show that children born small for gestational age are intellectually disadvantaged, but others do not. However, IQ testing in children is notoriously inaccurate. In the United Kingdom, researchers have followed over fourteen thousand full-term infants born in 1970, applying a variety of measures, including educational, employment and social success in later life. This study found that by the time they are sixteen years old, babies born small for gestational age are more likely to have been referred for special education. At age twenty-six, they are shorter in stature, have lower incomes and, compared with normal-weight babies, are less likely to have professional or managerial jobs.[5]

Programmed for life?

Now called gestational programming, we know that a low intake of essential nutrients during pregnancy changes the way a baby develops in the womb. Undernutrition can limit the ability of cells to divide, compromising the development of fetal organs. For example, in late pregnancy when organs are growing fastest, undernutrition permanently reduces kidney cell numbers. Since kidneys play a central role in regulating blood pressure, babies born small for gestational age are more likely to have problems controlling their blood pressure later, even in childhood.[6]

There are changes at the molecular level too—modifications to genes that alter how they function. The genes themselves are not changed but are "tagged" with tiny chemical markers that tell them when to work and when to stop working. The addition of these tags to genes is called epigenetics, from the Greek *epi,* meaning "on top of." Although all cells in a person's body contain the same set of genes, in different cell types genes are expressed differently—some are turned on, while others are turned off. Epigenetics is the reason a brain cell looks different from a heart cell or a skin cell.

Epigenetics controls how our genes interact with the environment. External factors like toxin exposure, infection and stress can all imprint genes. Once in place, epigenetic modifications can be passed down from one generation to the next. This interaction of genes and environment explains why one person may be constitutionally anxious or another may have a tendency to gain weight easily. It also explains why these tendencies are likely to be present in their children.

Both pre- and postnatal anxiety in the mother has a powerful influence on the developing baby's mental health. If a pregnancy is shrouded in apprehension and depression, this affects the way the baby's hippocampus develops. The hippocampus is an important part of the limbic system that regulates emotions and is strongly associated with memory, particularly long-term memory. If the anxiety continues after the baby is born, the negative effects on the baby's future mental health will be even more pronounced.

Finally, with this new understanding of the transmission of traits from one generation to another we can answer the age-old question, Which is more important, nature (genes) or nurture (epigenetics)? The answer is that both are critical. Prenatal epigenetic programming can influence personality, future risk of addictive behaviours, and the onset, progression and severity of chronic disease.

You are what your mother ate

However, all is not doom and gloom. We can intervene in this epigenetic transmission of disease risk. At least in animal studies, healthy nutrition before and during pregnancy can clear those epigenetic tags and wipe genes clean.[7] This is why pregnancy planning is so important. We really are what our mothers ate. And since the egg we developed from was formed when our mothers were themselves in utero, epigenetically we are also what our grandmothers ate!

Fathers and grandfathers also shoulder some responsibility for the health of future generations. For example, obesity in either the mother or the father can program a child for future obesity.[8] Whether our fathers smoked, survived a famine or fought through the harrowing experience of war can all imprint their genes, and that imprinting can be passed on to us, their offspring. We also know that what both our parents were exposed to during their own time in the womb—smoking, excess alcohol, stress, and toxins like mercury, herbicides and pesticides—can cause epigenetic changes that they can pass on to us.[9]

The health of a baby is also influenced by what mothers avoid. One example that has recently attracted attention is exposure to bisphenol A (BPA), a chemical found in many plastics. Prenatal and early childhood exposure to BPA has been linked to later chronic anxiety, depression and hyperactivity, especially in boys.[10] BPA is present in many household products, including food and drink containers and dental composites.[11] Until it was banned in many countries, many baby bottles contained BPA.

Too little or too much?

In developed countries, we are seeing signs that excessive calorie intake and unbalanced, unhealthy eating patterns are also a problem. Obesity and a high-fat diet during pregnancy and breastfeeding programs the baby not only for future obesity but also for increased vulnerability to mood disorders.[12] At the same time, the two essential dietary fats discussed in Chapter 2—the omega-3s and omega-6s—are typically unbalanced in Western diets. A high intake of the omega-6s in the absence of sufficient omega-3s compromises brain development.[13]

Many of the complications of pregnancy can be avoided with careful diet. Gestational diabetes, for example, not only affects the baby's growth rate and future risk of diabetes, but affects the mother's health too, increasing her risk of developing full-blown diabetes later. We know that the type and amount of carbohydrate eaten is important if you want to avoid excessive weight gain and diabetes. Repeatedly spiking blood glucose levels—eating a high glycemic load—leads to excessive weight gain, insulin resistance and gestational diabetes.[14]

Pregnant women want to avoid gestational diabetes, and should therefore avoid as much added sugar as possible and make sure that all grains are as unprocessed as possible. As we have seen, grains pulverized into flour can raise blood sugar as fast as a sugary drink. Vegetables and fruit generally have a low glycemic index and provide the steady supply of glucose the baby's developing brain needs. They are also packed full of fibre and phytochemicals. As we have seen, phytochemicals have major health benefits as antioxidants, antimicrobials and detoxifiers. These are carbohydrates that pack a major nutritional punch without causing hyperglycemia. A high intake in pregnancy may also help prevent childhood allergies.[15]

Why protein is important

Having suffered some pretty bad press over the years, protein is moving back to centre stage, its rightful place in a healthy pregnancy. The amino acids protein provides are the building blocks for every cell and tissue in the developing baby. They are also needed to make the hormones and neurotransmitters crucial for maintaining a healthy pregnancy. Protein is especially important in the last trimester of pregnancy to meet not only the needs of the growing baby, but also the needs of the mother, whose breasts and belly and internal organs must enlarge to accommodate her growing infant.

Since we can't store protein, we need a consistent, steady intake each day. This is important for someone with morning sickness, particularly the most severe form, *hyperemesis gravidarum*. After one to three days of unmet protein requirements, muscle will be broken down to provide the amino acids that diet is not supplying. For someone experiencing nausea during pregnancy I emphasize that at all costs protein needs must be met, and I usually recommend several protein shakes a day. These can be sipped slowly over the course of several hours, and are usually well tolerated.

Can you eat too much protein?

As pregnancy progresses, protein needs increase. The current recommendation suggests that 0.88 g of protein per kilogram of body weight meets the needs for protein in pregnancy—approximately 60 g a day for a 70 kg (150 lb.) woman. However, this recommendation is based on outdated methods of calculating protein requirements. Newer methods suggest that a protein intake of 1.22 g per kilogram of body weight is required for the first thirty weeks of pregnancy. This increases to 1.66 g for the remainder of the pregnancy—almost 50 per cent over the current recommendation.[16]

Despite evidence to the contrary, many articles in both the popular and medical press stubbornly insist that North Americans may eat too much protein, whereas surveys show that many of us eat too little, especially in pregnancy and old age. What *is* true is that North Americans eat too much protein at one meal—usually the evening meal—and that's a bad thing. Studies suggest that we can process only about 30 g of protein at one time. Since the excess cannot be stored, it must be converted into sugar and then into fat, a process that drains our micronutrient resources. In addition, more nitrogen waste must be removed from the blood, which puts a strain on the kidneys.

Current research suggests that it is important to spread your protein intake out over the course of the day.[17] In Chapter 14 we'll discuss how to get enough protein at each meal. Enough, but not too much.

The fats of life

Growing up close to the picturesque fishing port of Howth in North Dublin, we were lucky to have access to a wonderful variety of ocean-fresh fish and seafood. On Tuesdays and Thursdays the trawlers would return to the harbour for the fishermen to land their catch, and we were able to buy the fish straight off the boats. My mother was an excellent cook, and before long a delicious fish feast would appear on the table.

Back then, fish on Friday was the rule in Catholic households. For some of my friends who did not like fish, Friday dinner was the least popular meal of the week, but they had to eat it anyway. "It's food for the brain," their parents insisted. Call it instinctive nutrition, but those parents were right, although it would be several decades before scientists confirmed the link between fish consumption and brain health.

Omega-3 fats and the brain

As we saw in Chapter 3, two types of fats are essential: omega-3 and omega-6 fats. Two long-chain omega-3 fats—eicosapentaenoic acid (EPA) and docosahexaenoic acid (DHA)—found only in fish are important for the normal functioning of all body tissues. For the brain, the omega-3 fats take on a special significance. They form an integral part of the receptors for dopamine and serotonin, so a brain deprived of omega-3 fats will have difficulty utilizing these neurotransmitters.

Studies have shown that babies who received additional omega-3 fats through fish oil supplements during pregnancy sleep through the night earlier—a boon to parents.[18] Omega-3 fats are also important for the development of the eyes, because DHA is needed for retinal development. In animal studies, shortfalls of omega-3 fatty acids during pregnancy are linked to poorer vision that may not be reversible with dietary changes after birth.[19] Increased intake of omega-3 fatty acids during pregnancy also reduces the risk of postpartum depression in the mother.[20]

Our ancestors would have obtained essential fats by eating a shore-based diet, that is, one rich in fish and other seafood, bird's eggs, frogs and aquatic plants. In fish, the original source of EPA and DHA is marine algae, and these fats are therefore concentrated in fish that live off algae. Vegetarians can obtain DHA and EPA from algal oil supplements, although they are expensive. Flaxseed, canola and soybean oils do contain omega-3 fatty acids but not the long-chain DHA and EPA needed for brain development.

The problem with obtaining omega-3s from fish is that fish stocks have become contaminated with mercury and other pollutants. Low-level mercury exposure is neurotoxic, and exposure in pregnancy has been linked to a greater risk of attention deficit disorder. Pregnant women are therefore advised to limit seafood consumption to 340 g (two six-ounce servings) per week. This amount of fish will provide approximately 200 mg of DHA per day. However, higher amounts may be beneficial. A study in Mexican women found that supplements of 400 mg of DHA resulted in babies who weighed more at birth and had larger head circumferences—both factors that have been linked to higher IQ in childhood.[21] Most omega-3 supplements provide approximately 500 mg of DHA and 750 mg of EPA per serving.

An added bonus for those who don't like fish is that supplements don't usually taste fishy! The oil is distilled to remove any mercury or other pollutants, and this process removes the fish taste too. Most manufacturers add natural flavours like citrus or strawberry extract.

Choline: The forgotten fat

Choline, a fatty vitamin-like essential nutrient, is made in small amounts in the liver. It is often included with the B vitamins or referred to as "a B-like vitamin," but unlike folic acid, B6 or B12, most people have never heard of it. Choline is the building block for acetylcholine, the most abundant neurotransmitter in the body and the chemical that ferries messages between the brain and our muscles telling them to work. We can manufacture an amount sufficient for basic survival—for the smooth muscles that control our breathing and digestion, and cardiac muscle that controls heart function.

Acetylcholine is also known as the brain's "memory manager." It is critical for the formation of memories and for the development of verbal and logical reasoning. Consuming extra choline during pregnancy enhances attention span and spatial intelligence.[22] Spatial intelligence allows us to understand our world in three dimensions—what's up, what's down, in front or behind, and the difference between right and left. Poor spatial intelligence makes us clumsy and awkward and slow to react. For people with poor spatial intelligence, following directions or parking a car can be a challenge. They are unlikely to be chess champions or excel at mathematics.

The importance of choline was officially recognized only in 1998, when an adequate choline intake was established. An adequate intake is used when insufficient scientific evidence is available to set a recommended daily intake of a nutrient, based on estimates of what the average healthy person consumes. For women this is 425 mg a day and for men it is 550 mg. But average intakes are thought to be far below these levels.[23] There is also genetic variation in need for choline, so this estimate may not be optimal for everyone. During pregnancy and breastfeeding the mother's liver will increase its capacity to make choline, but despite this boost, demand usually exceeds the supply and body stores are depleted. Breastfeeding increases demand and further depletes tissue stores.

Where do we get choline?

Traditionally, liver and egg yolks were the two richest dietary sources of choline. Smaller amounts are present in milk and meat and in vegetable sources like peanuts and cauliflower. While liver is nutritious, there may be good reasons not to depend on it for choline intake during pregnancy. The liver is where drugs, hormones and environmental pollutants go for detoxification, and these toxins may be highly concentrated in the livers of animals raised with modern farming methods. If you enjoy eating liver and have access to an organic supply, then it is a healthy addition to any diet, especially during pregnancy. Three ounces of liver provides about 350 mg of choline.

Throughout human history, eggs have been a valued part of our diets.

At only seventy-five calories each, eggs contain 6 g of high-quality protein and a hefty dose of choline; one egg yolk can provide 125 mg (there is no choline in the egg white). In recent years we have been discouraged from eating eggs. Cholesterol-rich foods like egg yolks and seafood were thought to raise circulating blood cholesterol levels, a known risk for heart disease. But there is no evidence that the cholesterol that the doctor measures in our blood originates from our food—we make most of it ourselves. Removing cholesterol-rich foods from our diet has not been shown to help reduce blood levels of cholesterol.[24]

Can you turn stress genes off in pregnancy?

For most women, pregnancy is a magical time, filled with excitement and joyful anticipation. But unfortunately stress casts a shadow over some pregnancies. It might be the stress of an unexpected job loss or a sudden bereavement, or just the day-to-day stress of juggling a career and family life. In Canada, between 8 and 11 per cent of women go through pregnancy suffering from what psychiatrists call generalized anxiety disorder—pathological worry and uncontrollable anxiety about ordinary, everyday things. The trouble is that when the mother is under stress, so is her baby. As we have seen, babies exposed to high levels of anxiety during pregnancy have a heightened stress response, and are themselves vulnerable to lifelong depression and anxiety. No woman wants this for her baby, but most are reluctant to take medication during pregnancy for fear it may harm their unborn child.

Cornell University researchers have discovered a safe nutritional solution that appears to offer the baby some protection from maternal stress—extra choline. They studied twenty-six healthy women in the third trimester of pregnancy. Half were given diets containing approximately 480 mg of choline, a little more than official recommendations, while the others received 930 mg of choline, more than double current recommendations. Then researchers measured the stress hormone cortisol in blood samples taken from the mothers and their babies immediately after birth. The higher intake of choline did not alter the mothers' stress hormones. However, it significantly lowered those hormones in the babies.[25]

This higher intake of choline is difficult to obtain from diet without supplements. I encourage all pregnant women to eat at least one egg a day, preferably two, and organic liver once a week if they like it. But in addition I recommend extra choline supplements, described in Chapter 10. It makes me sad to see pregnancy cookbooks that suggest that egg-white omelettes make a good breakfast. While low-fat diets are desirable, too often low fat is interpreted as no fat. Unwittingly, many people who are conscientious about their diet have thrown the good fats out with the bad—the baby with the bathwater, so to speak.

What "eating for two" really means

While gaining too little weight during pregnancy is a concern, increasing the risk of premature delivery and low birth weight, the notion that pregnant women should be "eating for two" is a myth.

Excessive weight gain is linked to increased risk of complications in pregnancy and increases the likelihood that the baby will become an obese adult. It also strongly influences whether the mother will shed the extra pounds she has gained or remain overweight after the baby is born. Experts differ on the amount of extra calories needed during pregnancy. According to the U.S. Institute of Medicine, the baby is so small during the first trimester that no extra calories are needed, and an additional two to three hundred calories may be all the baby needs during the second and third trimesters.

However, some experts argue that extra calories may not be required at all. Researchers at Imperial College London have recently shown that conception triggers the release of special thyroid-like hormones that cause dramatic growth in the mother's intestines. This resizing of the mother's intestines helps her extract more energy from food, anticipating the energy needs of her growing baby.[26] And while so far the work has been mainly carried out in animal models, the researchers believe the same processes are at work in human pregnancies.

While a lot of extra calories may not be necessary when "eating for two," the need for vitamins and minerals certainly goes up. The next chapter looks at specific supplements that may be beneficial in pregnancy.

CHAPTER 9

Supplements and Pregnancy

Life is a flame that is always burning itself out, but it catches fire again every time a child is born.

GEORGE BERNARD SHAW

For a long time, a fetus was thought of as the "perfect parasite," siphoning off from its mother all the nourishment needed for its development. However, by the 1980s this idea was fading. As one review put it, "The fetus is not a 'perfect parasite'; maternal stores can be drawn upon for support but a limit exists as to the ability of the fetus to drain maternal supplies."[1]

In fact, both mother and baby suffer when the mother's intake of essential nutrients is inadequate. Although all nutrients are important for brain development, some appear to have greater effects in late pregnancy and infancy. These include protein, choline and the long-chain polyunsaturated fatty acids discussed in Chapter 8, iron, zinc, iodine and folate.[2] For the mother, deficiencies increase the risk of prolonged labour, high blood pressure, gestational diabetes and excessive bleeding before and after giving birth. For the baby, lack of key nutrients increases the risk of birth defects, type 1 diabetes and leukemia in childhood, and a host of psychiatric disorders—from learning disabilities like attention deficit and hyperactivity, to autism spectrum disorders and schizophrenia.[3]

On the positive side, providing these extra nutrients during pregnancy offers advantages to both the parents and the baby. As we saw in the previous chapter, babies of mothers who took fish oil while pregnant slept through the night earlier. And a higher consumption of choline-rich eggs or choline supplements lays the foundation for lifelong memory and learning abilities.[4]

Supplements needed for a healthy pregnancy

It is now clear that worldwide, intakes of vitamins and minerals are not sufficient for pregnancy. Supplementation is already recommended in low- and middle-income countries, especially for folic acid, iron, copper, zinc and iodine, since each of these nutrients is known to have an impact on neurological and intellectual development,[5] and intakes are generally below the recommended daily intake (RDI). However, even in high-income countries consumption of many essential nutrients does not meet recommended intakes. Even when they do, some experts argue that the RDIs themselves are too low for optimal fetal development and do not take into account individual variations in needs.[6] Take iron, for example, which is needed for proper brain development and hemoglobin production. Without iron, mitochondrial function is compromised and the axons of neurons are not properly myelinated. It is essential for the manufacture of serotonin and dopamine. The offspring of both animal and human females who were iron deficient while pregnant perform poorly on cognitive and behavioural tests.[7]

The daily requirement for iron varies considerably from one person to another: recent research has shown that someone with high needs may need forty times as much iron as someone with the lowest requirements.[8] Such diversity in daily requirements cannot possibly be accommodated by a one-size-fits-all approach. Fortunately, for decades now doctors have monitored iron needs during pregnancy, and they routinely check hemoglobin and ferritin, an indicator of body iron stores. Even in women with perfectly normal test results, a little extra iron is thought to be beneficial in pregnancy, and easily obtained from a prenatal multivitamin.

The folic acid story

The story of supplements in pregnancy is the story of folic acid. It begins in the 1920s. A young doctor, Lucy Wills, is researching macrocytic anemia, a type of blood disorder. In pursuit of her research she goes to India, where there is an exceptionally high incidence in female textile workers, especially when they are pregnant.

The fact that macrocytic anemia is more frequent in populations eating diets low in protein, fruit and vegetables leads her to suspect that a dietary deficiency might be involved. Experimentally, she can produce macrocytic anemia in rats by manipulating their diets. Moreover, she can cure the rats of their anemia with a yeast extract called Marmite, and she finds that Marmite works just as well for the pregnant textile workers. Later research shows that the protective factor in Marmite is folate, one of the B vitamins.

Fast-forward to the 1960s. Two U.K. researchers, Richard Smithells and Elizabeth Hibbard, are using urine analysis to test for folate deficiency. They notice that women who have given birth to a baby with spina bifida have test results suggestive of folate deficiency. Since they know folate plays a major role in cell division, they are concerned. Is it possible that folic acid deficiency is responsible for this devastating birth defect?

The word "folate" comes from *folium*, Latin for "leaf," since apart from yeast extracts like Marmite, leafy green vegetables are the richest dietary source. Once extracted from food, folate is unstable and difficult to work with. But in 1941 a synthetic version of folate, folic acid, becomes available, which is ideal for clinical trials. From the 1960s onwards multiple studies prove Smithells and Hibbard's hunch to be correct. Giving women folic acid before conception dramatically decreases the incidence of spina bifida.

Why does a shortage of folate in pregnancy have such devastating effects?

Normally, the nerve cells and fibres connecting the brain to the rest of the body are protected by the bony vertebrae of the spine. But if folate intake is low in pregnancy, the spine fails to form properly, leaving parts of the spinal cord unprotected and vulnerable to injury. Infants born with spina bifida—literally "split backbone"—may have significant nerve damage and partial or total paralysis of the lower limbs. Folic acid deficiency also causes other birth defects like cleft lip and palate, and congenital heart disease.

Today all women of childbearing age are encouraged to take folic acid supplements. And at least sixty countries around the world, including Canada and the United States, now fortify foods with folic acid.

But food fortification is not a complete solution. Taking folic acid as part of a multivitamin is better than taking folic acid alone, preventing approximately 92 per cent of these devastating birth defects.[9] Recent research suggests that spina bifida is also less common in mothers who have a high choline intake during pregnancy.[10]

Dynamic duo: Folic acid and vitamin B12

Of all the vitamins and minerals that work together, none cooperate more closely than the B vitamins, especially folic acid and vitamin B12. B12 is needed to metabolize folic acid into its active form, methyltetrahydrofolate. Imbalance of these two vitamins during pregnancy—that is, too little B12 relative to folic acid—is now known to have a detrimental effect on pregnancy outcomes. Babies exposed to this non-physiological balance are shorter, weigh less and have smaller head circumferences at birth.[11]

While the increased need for folate in pregnancy is met through folic acid supplementation or food fortification, its companion B12 is rarely given the same attention. Most prenatal multivitamins have up to 1 mg (1,000 µg) of folic acid but no more than 50 mg of B12. Since it is important to correct this huge imbalance, I always suggest additional B12.

Are most people B12 deficient?

While it is perfectly normal for newborns to cry when they are hungry, need a clean diaper or perhaps just want the physical comfort of a cuddle, a constantly crying baby generates a huge amount of anxiety and frustration in new parents. Dutch researchers looked at links between low blood levels of B12 in pregnant women and excessive crying. They defined "excessive" as crying for more than three hours a day. Although the mothers' blood level of folate was not linked to excessive crying, low B12 certainly was.[12]

B12 is found only in animal foods. Dairy products, eggs, meat, fish, poultry and shellfish are the best sources. Vegetarians and vegans are therefore at increased risk of B12 deficiency. To be absorbed from food, B12 must first attach to a protein called intrinsic factor, which is secreted in the stomach. For various reasons, some people don't make enough of this carrier protein. Crohn's disease, celiac disease or weight-loss surgery can also cause problems with B12 absorption.

To make intrinsic factor, stomach acid is needed, so taking antacids for digestive problems like reflux will block B12 absorption. Reflux is common in late pregnancy and often treated with antacids. Examples of drugs commonly used include proton pump inhibitors (PPIs) like Nexium and H2-receptor antagonists like Tagamet and Zantac. Metformin, a drug used to treat type 2 diabetes, also interferes with B12 absorption. So even when diets contain plenty of B12, there are obstacles to achieving B12 blood levels that balance the almost universally high blood levels of folic acid that are now common in countries with food fortification.

One way around problems with dietary B12 absorption is injections, but B12 lozenges are just as effective. When you suck these lozenges, the B12 they contain is absorbed into the bloodstream directly from the mouth.[13] No upper limit for B12 has been set for North America or Europe, since neither a high intake of B12 supplements nor high blood levels have any known toxicity.[14] I usually recommend a minimum of 1 mg (1,000 µg) daily in the lozenge form.

Zinc and copper

Zinc deficiency in the last trimester of pregnancy compromises brain growth. It can also alter hormones involved with the onset of labour, and zinc deficiency has been associated with increased risk of preterm birth.[15] Normal immune function depends on adequate zinc levels, and insufficient zinc increases the risk of infection in both mother and baby, another risk for preterm delivery. But be warned! Zinc has a narrow therapeutic window, meaning that there is only a small difference between doses that are necessary and beneficial and those that may be too high. Too much zinc can suppress immunity.

Copper is needed for blood vessel formation and heart health. It stabilizes collagen, the glue that binds our tissues together. It is needed for brain development and for the production of energy by mitochondria. Zinc and copper compete with one another for absorption and need to be taken in balance. A well-formulated prenatal multivitamin usually contains balanced amounts of both these pregnancy-essential trace minerals: approximately 15 mg of zinc and 2 mg of copper.

Iodine, thyroid function and pregnancy

Iodine's major role is to make the thyroid hormone, thyroxine. Iodine deficiency therefore compromises thyroid function. This can affect fertility, since low thyroid function suppresses the release of an egg at ovulation. Worldwide, iodine deficiency is one of the leading preventable causes of mental retardation. One investigation found that children whose mothers were iodine deficient had IQ scores 6.9 to 10.2 points lower when compared with the offspring of mothers with good iodine status.[16]

One obvious sign of poor iodine status is goitre—a painful swelling in the neck due to enlargement of the thyroid gland. Iodine deficiency was once common in many areas of North America, especially around the Appalachians, Great Lakes and northwestern regions of the United States, a region that became known as the goitre belt. After iodine was added to table salt, from the 1920s onwards, the incidence of goitre fell from about 30 per cent to under 2 per cent of the population. However, today many people avoid added table salt because of fears that it will increase blood pressure.

The daily requirement for iodine increases by approximately 50 per cent during pregnancy. Increasing salt intake by that amount is not desirable, so supplementing with iodine is therefore essential. Prenatal multivitamins usually contain 150 mg of iodine, which is plenty.

Developing bones and vitamin D

On my office wall hangs a framed advertisement dated 1928, urging mothers to supplement babies and children with cod liver oil in case they don't get enough sunshine. It helps baby's bones and teeth develop properly and prevents infection, the advert says. And it's good for expectant and nursing mothers too, protecting their teeth and bones from deterioration.

For some reason—probably because it tasted awful—we stopped using cod liver oil, assuming we could obtain enough vitamin D from food and sun exposure. As we have seen, it is difficult to get enough vitamin D from food, even when it is fortified. More recently we started to warn people not to expose themselves to the sun for fear of skin cancer. The result has been a catastrophic rise in vitamin D deficiency.

The re-emergence of rickets

Rickets is the most extreme form of vitamin D deficiency. To build strong bones, calcium and phosphorus are needed, but to absorb these two minerals we need vitamin D. Bones with rickets are soft, brittle and prone to fractures. Bowed or bandy legs, skull malformations, curved spines, protruding or "pigeon" chests and misshapen pelvic bones are all hallmarks of rickets. Rickets is fatal if not treated. That's because calcium is needed for more than strong bones—it is needed to keep the heart beating.

Today we are seeing a resurgence of rickets. From North America to Australia and even sun-rich regions like the Middle East, a disease that had once been stopped in its tracks is re-emerging.[17] "The babies are irritable, they look unwell, they're not gaining weight, not growing in length and their legs aren't straight," says Dr. Leanne Ward, a pediatric endocrinologist at the Children's Hospital of Eastern Ontario in Ottawa. Dr. Ward is heading a two-year study to see how widespread the incidence of rickets in Canada is.

In the United Kingdom, researchers have been able to identify rickets in babies before they are born. A special 3D ultrasound can detect inappropriate bone development as early as nineteen weeks of pregnancy, even in women who are only borderline vitamin D deficient.[18] If these babies then face a difficult or traumatic birth, their fragile bones will suffer fractures. If the fractures are discovered while the baby is still in hospital, the condition is called transient idiopathic rickets. The babies are given a large dose of vitamin D and appear to recover.

Miscarriage of justice?

But once an infant with undetected rickets goes home, even normal everyday movements like dressing and undressing may cause a fracture. Vitamin D deficiency can also cause unusual bruising as well as bleeding into the baby's brain or eyes. The tragedy is that these symptoms, especially when they occur together with fractures, are generally assumed to be signs of child abuse.

In 2012 two young British parents, Karrissa Cox and Richard Carter, noticed blood in the mouth of their six-week-old son after feeding him. Concerned, they rushed to the hospital, where the baby was found to have minor bruises and also some fractures on X-ray. The parents were charged with child abuse, and social services removed the baby to foster care. Cox and Carter were devastated. They knew they had not harmed their baby. Fortunately for them, all babies in the United Kingdom have blood taken five days after birth and stored as a spot on a card—the Guthrie card. When the baby's Guthrie spot was checked, it showed severe vitamin D deficiency, which was the cause of the fractures and bleeding.

However, in the meantime, the local authorities had allowed the baby to be legally adopted. "We took our child to the hospital seeking help and they stole our baby from us" was the heartbreaking comment from the young couple after being exonerated by the courts. Now they are seeking the return of their child, but since the baby was legally adopted it will be an uphill battle. As their defence lawyer said after their court appearance, "These innocent parents have been spared a criminal conviction and prison sentence for a crime they never committed. Their life sentence is that they are likely never to see their baby again." This is just one of a number of cases that have recently come to light, which probably represent just the tip of the iceberg.

Whose responsibility is it to make certain that cases like this are prevented in future? Is it the job of the parents? Or is it the responsibility of the various medical practitioners and public health agencies advising women during pregnancy? One scientific paper suggests that vitamin D supplementation during pregnancy should have the same priority as any other public health intervention designed to protect the interests of the unborn child. It is simply a basic human right.[19]

Brain development and vitamin D

At birth, rats born to vitamin D-deficient mothers have profound alterations in their brains. They have impaired attention processing and are at increased risk of psychosis and schizophrenia-like behaviour.[20] Spanish researchers who had measured the vitamin D levels in the blood of two thousand women during the first and second trimesters of pregnancy found that, at fourteen months, the children of mothers who had 25-hydroxyvitamin D levels less than 50 nmol/L (20 ng/mL) scored lower on tests of mental and physical skills.[21] Commenting on the Spanish study, neonatologist Dr. Valencia Walker, MD, from Mattel Children's Hospital, UCLA, said, "This study proves that D matters, and that pregnant women should not be vitamin D deficient."

Autism spectrum disorders are increasingly diagnosed in many developed countries. In the United States, about one in sixty-eight children is identified with autism spectrum disorder, almost double the incidence seen in 2002.[22] Whether this rise is due to increased incidence or increased diagnosis is debated. Either way, the numbers are alarming for a disease that was once thought to be extremely rare. The question that really needs to be addressed is, Why do we have so many children with autism spectrum disorders?

Some scientists believe that vitamin D deficiency plays a role. A recent review of eleven studies found a definite association between decreased maternal vitamin D levels in pregnancy and increased risk for autism in the offspring.[23] It is tempting, therefore, to draw a parallel between the apparent rise in autism and growing concern about declining blood levels of vitamin D worldwide.[24]

Samantha's story

Kimberly was a young woman I worked with before she started a family. Because she played a lot of ice hockey, I was concerned that she might have low reserves of some nutrients. She sweated intensely when playing, and both sweating and strenuous physical exertion deplete nutrients. And so she embarked on the usual supplement program I recommend for pregnancy.

In due course Kimberly became pregnant, and nine months later Tara was born. Tara was a sweet baby, but as she grew into a toddler, worrying signs of ADHD began to appear. She was unable to sit still for stories or games. At daycare she could not follow rules or routines. She constantly climbed on furniture or crawled under it. Although there was no formal diagnosis, Tara's parents suspected the presence of ADHD in both their families.

Several years later baby brother Michael arrived, and a few years after that, Samantha was born. In temperament these two younger children were as different from Tara as chalk from cheese. Both were easygoing, slept through the night from an early age and showed no signs of behaviour typical of ADHD. One day, Kimberly and her husband arrived at my office for their appointments, bringing fourteen-month-old Samantha with them.

Since both parents liked to sit in on each other's appointments, in total they would be in my office for two hours, and I was concerned about having a small child in the office for more than a quick visit. I needn't have worried. For a few moments Samantha fussed. Then she climbed off her mother's lap, toddled round to my side of the desk, raised her arms and said, "Up." I lifted her onto my knee, and there she stayed contentedly for the rest of our session. From time to time she fiddled with the keys in my desk drawer, but mostly she sat still and listened to what I was saying, cocking her head to one side and looking alternately from her parents to me. It was almost as if she were taking in everything we were discussing. Intrigued, her mother pulled out her cellphone and snapped a picture of us.

I kept that photograph on my desktop for months. It reminded me that toddlers can be calm and patient and don't need to become frustrated in strange or restrictive environments. Her older sister could not have coped. She would have been fidgeting, running around the office and interrupting our discussion all the time. The appointment would have been impossible.

If only we'd known

All three babies had received similar diets in utero, and Kimberly had taken *almost* the same supplements while pregnant. But shortly after Tara was born, I became aware that the standard recommendations for vitamin D during pregnancy did not take into account individual genetic needs or the baseline vitamin D status of the mother, and might therefore be inadequate. So I started testing vitamin D.

To my surprise Kimberly's blood test came back low, even though she had been taking 2,000 IU (50 mg) daily for some years. I increased her vitamin D, and by the time she got pregnant with Michael and Samantha she had been taking 4,000 IU (100 mg) for some time. Was it just chance that the personalities of Michael and Samantha were so very different from Tara's, or was increasing Kimberly's vitamin D a factor? Since then, research has shown that inadequate vitamin D in pregnancy may indeed play a role in the development of ADHD.[25]

When Tara was ten years old her diagnosis was sadly changed to autism spectrum disorder. Current research suggests that this too may be linked to insufficient vitamin D during an otherwise healthy pregnancy.[26] This hypothesis is strengthened by the finding that mothers with dark skin who live in northerly countries like Sweden or Canada are at increased risk of having an autistic child.[27] Both darker skin tones and living at higher latitudes are risk factors for vitamin D deficiency.

Vitamin D deficiency certainly cannot take sole responsibility for the development of autism. Other factors, including genetic predisposition and exposure to environmental pollutants, are also thought to play a role. However, animal experiments show that orderly brain development is dependent on the presence of adequate vitamin D levels during pregnancy and early childhood.[28] Since it is simple to test for deficiency, I believe that all women wishing to become pregnant need to have their

vitamin D status checked and make sure that any shortfall is treated
with vitamin D supplements.

Like her siblings, Tara is highly intelligent, but her behaviour is
exhausting for her parents and teachers. She will require very special
support if she is to achieve her full intellectual potential.

What about vitamin D supplements?

Vitamin D is cheap and supplements are readily available. But how do we
know how much to take? What is the supplement equivalent of a healthy
daily dose of summer sun? Because of genetic variations, the same amount
of supplemental vitamin D may give dramatically different blood levels in
different individuals. As an editorial in one medical journal put it, "The
unpredictable relationship between vitamin D intake and blood levels
makes it difficult to recommend a standard supplement dose and supports
incorporating measurements of blood levels into recommendations."[29]

Surveys suggest that at least 25 per cent of white-skinned Canadians
have blood levels below the minimum cut-off point for bone health (50
nmol/L or 20 ng/mL), and this increases to 60 per cent among nonwhites.[30]
Remember, the darker your skin tone the more difficult it is to make vitamin D from sunshine. Studies have shown that taking the upper limit for
vitamin D—4,000 IU daily—throughout pregnancy is safe, and may reduce
the incidence of complications.[31] Ideally, a blood test should be done
after three months to make sure that this intake is sufficient to raise blood
levels into the reference range, which is 75–250 nmol/L in Canada and
30–100 ng/mL in the United States. Apart from the baby's health, good
blood levels of vitamin D during pregnancy may prevent postpartum
depression in the mother.[32]

Other nutritional needs in pregnancy

All the essential nutrients are needed for the growth and development
of a baby. Even though it is possible to point the finger at deficiencies
of certain key nutrients, the absence of any one of them would be likely
to have a detrimental effect on pregnancy outcomes.

Many couples busy with their careers delay trying to become pregnant until their thirties and forties and then have difficulty conceiving. Researchers believe vitamin E deficiency may contribute to this falling fertility. Vitamin E was originally named "the fertility vitamin" because of its essential role in normal reproduction. In the early days of vitamin research it was found that rats deprived of this vitamin became sterile. A U.S. study found that 93 per cent of twenty- to thirty-year-olds and 81 per cent of those over thirty had suboptimal vitamin E status.[33]

Adequate calcium intake may reduce the incidence of preterm delivery, and a daily intake of 1,000 mg is recommended before and during pregnancy and while breastfeeding. This amount is not difficult to obtain from diet, so supplements may not be necessary.

As we saw previously, one role of magnesium is to work in cooperation with calcium in the normal process of muscle contraction and relaxation. The efficient working of the heart, skeletal muscle, and the smooth muscle cells that control the lungs, the bladder and the gastrointestinal tract depend on this fine balance. Any calcium you take either as supplements or from diet should therefore be balanced carefully with magnesium. In the next chapter you will see how to calculate your intake of calcium to make sure you're getting enough but not too much, as well as how to balance it with your intake of magnesium.

An imbalance of magnesium relative to calcium is easy to detect since low magnesium usually produces characteristic symptoms, including leg cramps, fatigue and restless sleep. Shortness of breath and frequency of urination can also signal an imbalance. Dyspepsia—discomfort, bloating or a feeling of fullness with very little intake of food, as well as heartburn or regurgitation of food—may also signal magnesium needs. One uncomfortable indication for magnesium needs is increasing constipation during pregnancy. Taken correctly, magnesium can be very helpful for reflux and constipation. Using magnesium to treat these two conditions is accepted by mainstream medicine as standard care, although the evidence from well-designed clinical trials is limited.[34]

Vitamin C and pregnancy

Vitamin C is needed to make collagen, the most abundant molecule in the body after water. Collagen makes up a quarter of our entire body protein and gives strength and elasticity to skin, muscles, tendons and ligaments. About 80 per cent of pregnant women end up with stretch marks, or striae—those raised, white, scar-like wavy lines on the belly and upper thighs. These are a sign of disturbances in collagen production and a failure to meet the increased needs for collagen production as pregnancy progresses and belly skin expands.[35]

While stretch marks might be considered simply cosmetic and of little health importance, a more serious consequence of inadequate collagen production is the preterm or early rupture of the amniotic sac that surrounds and protects the fetus in the womb. Premature rupture of membranes is a leading cause of preterm birth. Blood levels of vitamin C decrease over the course of pregnancy, and a significant link has been shown between lower plasma vitamin C and premature rupture of membranes.[36] As with vitamin D, the amount of vitamin C from diet or in supplements is not a good predictor of what blood level of vitamin C will be achieved.

Children of our time?

There is growing evidence that pregnant women worldwide are deficient in critical fats necessary for the brain health of the developing child, and deficiency of the omega-3 fat DHA is also linked to preterm birth. In the United States, there are calls for supplementation of 600 mg of DHA daily for all pregnant women to prevent premature births. It has been estimated that this intervention could shave US$6 billion a year off health care costs, never mind prevent a lot of heartache.[37]

A Child of Our Time is a BBC documentary series that followed twenty-five children from their birth in 2000 to 2013. In one program, two young boys are shown with dramatically different emotional problems. James is out of control. His parents are faced with daily outbursts of anger and aggression. At school he is constantly in trouble for fighting—punching and kicking other children, and lashing out at everything and anything that frustrates him. Ruben's problems are different. He isn't a happy child. Uncommunicative with his parents and teachers, he has few friends. Neither of the boys is doing well at school.

A Child of Our Time documents what happens when both boys are given a daily supplement of fish oil. Over the course of the program we see a remarkable transformation in both children—changes that are as dramatic as they are inspiring. Three months after beginning the supplements, James can happily play with other children. He no longer fights or grabs other children's toys. He is calm and friendly. And the changes for Ruben are no less profound. He has blossomed—we see him chattering away with newfound friends and interacting well with his teacher. He no longer seems sad and isolated.

While we have no firm evidence that it was the fish oil that was instrumental in making these changes, this documentary seemed to hold out some hope that it's never too late to make up for dietary shortfalls that may have occurred during pregnancy. The documentary simply confirms what other research studies have shown: if our children have missed out before birth, we can certainly do something about it later on.

But how much better it would be if these nutritional needs were met right from conception.

CHAPTER 10

Prenatal Planning: A Checklist

Calvin: Dad, how do people make babies?
Dad: Most people just go to Sears, buy the kit, and follow the assembly instructions.
Calvin: I came from Sears??
Dad: No, you were a blue light special at K-Mart. Almost as good and a lot cheaper.

BILL WATTERSON,
Calvin and Hobbes

We have seen the evidence that nutrition in pregnancy can change the way genes work—changes that in turn affect the intellectual development and physical health of a baby for its entire life. Moreover, these changes can be inherited. This fact essentially makes future parents the de facto guardians of our gene pool and the health of future generations. A daunting prospect, and one that seems like a huge responsibility.

At the same time, the wealth of knowledge we have gained in the past few decades is exciting, and empowers tomorrow's mothers and fathers to take charge. They have opportunities to shape the future in ways their own parents could never have imagined. We can make better babies! Or more correctly, we can make it possible for the next generation of children to achieve their full physical and mental potential. Although Mother Nature undoubtedly has more secrets to reveal about what constitutes the perfect pregnancy diet, we know enough now to suggest multiple nutritional ways to promote brain development.

And it's never too early to start. Studies show that a woman's pre-pregnancy diet may be just as important as how she eats while pregnant. Supplements undoubtedly have a role to play too, especially since inadequate intakes of many micronutrients are widespread even in wealthy countries like Canada.[1] And even if you are not planning a pregnancy any time soon, improving your diet can only have a positive impact on your health, by increasing your energy levels, speed of mental processing, mood, focus and concentration.

A growing body of research suggests that the father's health at the time of conception affects the future physical and mental well-being of the baby.[2] So men may also want to up their game, nutritionally speaking, and carefully consider their responsibilities in preparing for parenthood.

Twelve evidence-based steps to a healthy pregnancy

1. Get into shape. Make sure that your body mass index (BMI) is in the normal range. Being underweight makes it more difficult to get pregnant in the first place and increases the risk of early miscarriage and preterm birth.[3]

Being overweight is not good either, increasing the risk of complications like gestational diabetes and pre-eclampsia, a serious disorder of late pregnancy characterized by high blood pressure and kidney problems.[4] And if either parent is overweight or obese, the child too is more likely to struggle with weight problems—an unintended legacy. Obesity (BMI ≥35) in both parents can influence their offspring's development too. Compared to children of normal-weight parents, those whose parents are both obese may have delayed development of fine motor and social skills.[5]

But it is never a good idea to go on a crash diet. Extreme diets are difficult to implement healthily and often severely restrict the amount of essential nutrients and phytochemicals consumed.[6] Crash dieters usually put weight back on quicker than those who follow a healthy diet and so may be vulnerable to excess weight gain in pregnancy. Nor is it sensible to try to increase low body weight by overindulging in high-calorie junk food. This might increase your weight but could magnify nutritional inadequacies.

If you have a history of eating disorders—either anorexia or bulimia—it is extremely important that you have been fully recovered for long enough to rebuild your nutritional stores. A long history of food restriction means your nutritional reserves are likely to be low, and a baby draws on these reserves to grow and develop. Drastically restricting food intake during pregnancy can be catastrophic for the developing baby.[7]

Ideally, I recommend at least one year on a healthy diet and supplement regime before attempting to conceive. Make sure you feel able to cope emotionally with the changing body shape and size that inevitably accompanies a healthy pregnancy, and get professional psychological support if you need it.

2. Start taking a prenatal multivitamin and mineral supplement.

Substantial research supports the regular use of multivitamins, rather than single nutrients like folic acid or vitamin D, to ensure a healthy pregnancy.[8] According to one report, "Micronutrient deficiencies are known to interact and greater benefit is achieved by multiple rather than single-nutrient supplementation."[9]

Many generic prenatal multivitamin and mineral supplements contain the recommended amount of folic acid but negligible amounts of the other B vitamins. We have seen that the B vitamins are interdependent and need to be taken in balance and together. Look for a supplement containing at least ten times the recommended daily intake (RDI) for all the B vitamins, if possible in their activated form. B vitamins normally require conversion by the liver so they can be absorbed and utilized, a task many of us do not do very effectively. With activated (or coenzyme) forms of B vitamins, the liver's work has been done for you, and the B vitamins can be used right away. A knowledgeable health professional or good health food store should be able to direct you to a suitable product.

Make sure that the prenatal supplement you are taking contains a minimum of 15 mg of zinc, 25–30 mg of iron and 150 µg of iodine. There is growing concern that iodine intake in North American women planning to get pregnant is suboptimal.[10] Fathers-to-be will also benefit from taking a daily multivitamin, since multivitamins improve both female and male fertility.[11]

3. Take additional B12. Although a prenatal multivitamin will contain ample folic acid, it is unlikely to offer sufficient B12. Remember that folic acid and B12 need to be balanced for optimal pregnancy outcomes. And as we have seen, B12 can be difficult to absorb, so some individuals may not benefit from what is present in their multivitamin. Taking B12 lozenges that you suck, or drops that you place under your tongue, overcomes any problem with absorption, since the B12 is absorbed directly into the bloodstream from the mouth.

Take B12 in its active form—methylcobalamin—available in most good pharmacies and health food stores. The folic acid we are commonly exposed to in diet and supplements can usually be offset by 1 mg (1,000 µg) of B12 taken once a day. This intake, although many times higher than the RDI, is safe in pregnancy—no upper limits have been set either for the amount of B12 you take or blood levels of B12, and no toxicity has ever been reported.

4. Increase omega-3 fats with fish oil. As we have seen, babies whose mothers took fish oil supplements during pregnancy slept through the night earlier. They also had better eye development and sharper vision.[12] When evaluated at two years of age, their scores for eye-hand coordination were higher and they were less clumsy as toddlers.

Although eating fatty fish rich in omega-3 fatty acids twice a week is recommended during pregnancy, research suggests that this does not supply enough of the critical EPA and DHA fats so important for optimal brain development. But increasing fish intake beyond the recommended two servings increases the risk of overexposure to mercury and other environmental pollutants, which may be detrimental to a developing baby's brain, so fish oil supplements are the safest and most reliable way to go. Read the label to make sure the supplement you use is certified free of heavy metals and other pollutants.

Because it takes time to increase the body's store of fats, I advise taking a fish oil supplement for at least three months prior to pregnancy. For vegetarians who prefer not to take fish oil, algal oil is a reliable alternative. Aim to consume approximately 500 mg of DHA with 750 mg of EPA daily. Rather than a handful of capsules, I generally suggest the oil itself in liquid form. This can be stirred into food like yogurt or unsweetened apple sauce for more consistent absorption.

This delicate fat is easily damaged. Store opened bottles in the fridge, and follow the manufacturer's recommendations for best-by date after opening. Do not add to hot food. Many people like to put their fish oil into a morning smoothie. This is an excellent way to take it since the fat increases the absorption of phytochemicals from the fruits and vegetables. But stir the oil in *after* making the smoothie—whizzing it up in the blender will damage it.

5. Eat a low-fat diet. But remember that low fat does not mean *no* fat. Every meal needs to contain some fat to help the body absorb phytochemicals and fat-soluble vitamins. Also remember that when it comes to fats, there are good and bad fats. Trans fats or partially hydrogenated fats found in processed and deep-fried foods have a negative impact on healthy brain development. A high consumption of trans fats may also affect fertility. In men, a diet high in trans fats can reduce sperm count.[13]

Both parents-to-be should avoid cookies, chips and other prepackaged convenience foods as well as deep-fried fast foods. In addition to a fish oil supplement, focus on healthy fats like olive oil, avocados, nuts and nut butters and organic coconut oil. Make sure to include small amounts of one of these good fats with each meal or snack.

6. Keep blood sugar under control. To avoid gestational diabetes and programming a baby for future weight problems, you need to watch your sugar and starch intake.[14] Try to cut out all added sugar and make sure that all grains are wholegrain. And remember, you want them to be as unprocessed as possible, since even whole grains will spike blood sugar when ground finely into flour.

Try limiting your intake of starchy foods like bread, rice and pasta to one serving per meal. A serving of bread is one slice, and a serving of rice, pasta or potatoes is half a cup, cooked. Scrap fruit juice in favour of whole fruit since juice is a very concentrated source of sugar. For example, an eight-ounce glass of orange juice can contain the equivalent of ten teaspoons of sugar—the same as a can of Coke.

Sugar-sweetened drinks really have no place in a healthy diet. If you cannot live without your daily can of soda, zero-calorie versions are available sweetened with stevia, a natural sweetener made from the leaves of a plant and used in South America and Asia for centuries. At present it seems to be the safest available zero-calorie sweetener.

7. Make ten servings of vegetables and fruit your daily target.

If you are not crazy about vegetables and haven't been getting the ten daily servings needed for optimal health, now is an excellent time to start. Fruits and vegetables provide the constant supply of glucose that a baby's developing brain needs. This steady input of glucose benefits the mother too and helps to prevent "baby brain"—the pregnancy-induced brain fog that many women complain of during and after pregnancy.

Fruits and vegetables are packed full of fibre and phytochemicals. As we have seen, phytochemicals have major health benefits—as antioxidants, antimicrobials and detoxifiers. These are the carbohydrates you really need, since they pack a major nutritional punch without causing swings in blood sugar. Switching to a "veggie-centric" diet where vegetables are a major component of every meal will help you achieve the ten daily servings. A high intake of phytochemicals during pregnancy can reduce the risk of childhood allergies.[15]

Eat as wide a variety of fruits, vegetables, herbs and spices as you can. This may make all the difference between having a child who happily eats their vegetables and a picky eater. Children's preferences for new foods introduced during weaning are influenced by the flavours and aromas that they experience while still in their mother's womb and, after birth, in breast milk.[16]

8. Consider choline. As we have already seen, extra choline in pregnancy enhances spatial intelligence and short-term working memory in the offspring, and the benefits appear to be lifelong, extending even into old age. Because a baby's demand for choline is high, it is best to start increasing your intake well before getting pregnant.

Egg yolks are a traditional dietary source of choline, and eating one to two eggs a day should not affect cholesterol levels.[17] If you don't like eggs or are allergic to them, you can use supplements. Lecithin, which is frequently used as an emulsifier in foods, comes from soy and is rich in choline. It can be purchased either as capsules or granules to sprinkle on food. One tablespoon provides approximately 2.5 grams of choline, well short of the tolerable upper intake level of 3.5 grams per day.

Choline is designated GRAS, which stands for "generally regarded as safe." This means there are no scientific concerns about its overuse. I usually recommend achieving an intake of about 1,000 mg daily, approximately the amount used in the pregnancy study from Cornell University discussed in Chapter 8.

9. Check vitamin D. Low levels of vitamin D circulating in blood are associated with increased risk of early miscarriage,[18] and as we saw in Chapter 9, very low levels can result in in utero rickets. Low levels increase the risk of Caesarean births, pre-eclampsia and gestational diabetes. There are also increasing concerns that low vitamin D in pregnancy increases vulnerability to autism.[19]

Blood levels of vitamin D take a while to increase after supplements are begun, climbing slowly over a three-month period before levelling off at any particular dose. Start taking 4,000 IU daily. This is the upper limit for anyone from the age of nine on and has been shown not only to be safe in pregnancy but to reduce the risk of pregnancy complications.[20] Blood levels above 100 nmol/L (40 ng/mL) have recently been shown to be optimal for preventing attention deficit hyperactivity disorder in children.[21] After three months, check your blood levels and, if they are still inadequate, work with your doctor to gradually increase your intake.

For maximum absorption remember to take vitamin D with food, preferably the largest meal of the day.

10. Balance calcium and magnesium. Calcium is critically important for the baby's developing bones and neurological health. If you don't consume enough, your own bones and teeth can liberate their calcium to meet the developing baby's needs. To avoid future dental problems and osteoporosis, make sure you get 1,000 mg daily. This includes calcium from diet and supplements, so don't forget the calcium in your multivitamin—some prenatal multivitamins contain 400 mg or more.

It is not difficult to obtain the remainder of your calcium requirement from diet, especially if you eat dairy products such as milk, cheese and yogurt. A thumb-sized serving of hard cheese, for example, will give you 200 mg. Dairy substitutes like almond milk are frequently fortified with extra calcium. Check the label. You can easily find out if your daily calcium intake is adequate by using one of the many online calcium calculators.[22] Try to keep your intake of calcium-rich foods similar from day to day, and avoid excessive intake.

Magnesium deficiency is widespread among women of childbearing age. In animal studies a low intake of magnesium in pregnancy prevents proper development of the placenta and reduces fetal growth.[23] Although people vary in their need for magnesium, a blood test won't help you decide whether you are getting enough. This is because serum magnesium is tightly controlled to regulate heart rate. By the time blood levels are low you could be seriously deficient.[24]

But you don't need a blood test to tell if you need more magnesium— there are very characteristic physical signs and symptoms related to how calcium and magnesium work together. As previously discussed, calcium is needed for muscles to contract, but they can't relax again if you are short of magnesium. Signs of imbalance between these two essential minerals include leg cramps and restless legs, shortness of breath and increased frequency of urination, especially at night. Gastrointestinal disturbances like constipation and reflux are further evidence you may be low in magnesium.[25] Many of these symptoms can become problems during pregnancy and reflect the need for more magnesium as pregnancy progresses.

The balance of calcium and magnesium is easily upset, especially if you go overboard on calcium-rich foods like milk. Most prenatal multivitamins contain approximately 100 mg of magnesium. The upper limit for magnesium supplements—that is, the amount that women aged nineteen and older can take without side effects—is set at 350 mg a day, with no increase for pregnancy or during breastfeeding. For some women this may be enough, but for many it is not.

The best form of magnesium to take is an amino-acid-bound form like magnesium glycinate. Take 100 mg every night before bed for sleep and to prevent leg cramps. Or, since individual needs for magnesium vary, you can personalize your own magnesium intake by following the method outlined in Chapter 15. It is best to do this under the supervision of a knowledgeable doctor or other health care practitioner.

11. Increase intake of antioxidant vitamins. The antioxidant vitamins are vitamin A, beta-carotene, vitamin C and vitamin E. Vitamin A is absolutely essential for the growth and development of a baby, especially for eye development. Too much vitamin A in pregnancy is not desirable, however, and most multivitamins limit the amount of vitamin A to 4,000 IU (1,200 mg). However, we can make vitamin A from beta-carotene, which is plentiful in orange and red fruits and vegetables. Beta-carotene is perfectly safe in pregnancy because your body will convert only the amount it needs to vitamin A. But you need other cofactors, particularly zinc and vitamin C, to do this efficiently.

While your diet can provide ample beta-carotene, it is helpful to supplement with extra vitamins C and E as a multivitamin is unlikely to contain optimal amounts of these two vitamins. Vitamin C is needed to manufacture collagen, the most abundant molecule in the body after water. Disruption of collagen production can lead to stretch marks and varicose veins, two common consequences of pregnancy. Collagen is the main supportive molecule in the amniotic sac—a tough membranous bag of waters in which your developing baby floats during pregnancy. Low plasma levels of vitamin C are seen in women whose membranes rupture prematurely.[26]

As an antioxidant vitamin, E protects the fats of the brain, including

DHA. Surveys suggest that roughly 90 per cent of North Americans do not meet recommended intakes of vitamin E. Take full-spectrum vitamin E, which combines all eight forms of vitamin E found in nature. Vitamin E and fish oil supplements together are thought to be important to reduce the risks of neurodevelopmental disorders like autism.[27] In couples being treated for unexplained infertility, a combination of vitamin E, vitamin C and beta-carotene was shown to decrease the time it took to get pregnant.[28]

12. Watch your protein intake. Protein has a major structural role to play in all body tissues, and is also needed to make the enzymes, hormones and neurotransmitters that keep our bodies functioning. Recent studies have shown that the current recommendation for protein in pregnancy of 0.88 g per kilogram of body weight per day is inadequate and seriously underestimates needs; 1.22 g per kilogram of body weight is required in early pregnancy and 1.66 in late pregnancy.[29] This amount translates into 25–35 g of protein at each meal for most mothers-to-be, depending on body weight.

Vegetarians, especially vegans, need to be particularly careful to get sufficient good-quality protein before and during pregnancy. Most vegetable sources of protein are incomplete—that is, they do not contain all nine essential amino acids. Absence or inadequate intake of any one amino acid can impair growth of the fetus during pregnancy. While three to four ounces of fish, chicken or lean beef can provide 25 g of protein for less than 200 calories, consuming the same amount of protein from almond or peanut butter would take seven tablespoons at approximately 650 calories. To consume 25 g of protein from black beans, you would need to eat one and a half typical fifteen-ounce cans at a cost of about 500 calories.

Meeting these higher requirements for protein from vegetarian sources can mean consuming unrealistically large amounts of food, and possibly overconsumption of calories and inappropriate weight gain. At the end of this book you'll find a list of some commonly consumed protein-rich foods from both animal and vegetable sources. Check the many websites that list protein sources for the protein content of your favourite foods, and make sure that before and during pregnancy your protein intake is optimal.

PART 4

Making Brains Last a Lifetime

CHAPTER 11

The Learning Brain: Diet and Academic Success

I am always doing that which I cannot do, in order that I may learn how to do it.

PABLO PICASSO

A hungry child can't learn. This is the main reason most developed countries have had school meal programs in place since the early twentieth century. But despite government-issued nutritional guidelines for school cafeterias, standard school fare is often the opposite of healthy—high in sugar, fat and starchy carbohydrates, and low in vegetables and fruit. The abysmal choices are usually blamed on the limited budgets schools have to work with.

While in the White House, First Lady Michelle Obama tried to raise awareness and to get parents to speak up on behalf of children: "We as parents need to be leading the conversation about kids' health in this country . . . when naysayers claim that we just can't afford to serve our kids healthy food, it's up to us as parents to push back and say, 'We can't afford not to give our kids nutritious food.'"

Even when schools do limit the amount of calories and sugar in the cafeteria, and ban pop and candy-dispensing machines, they don't necessarily provide healthy alternatives. In any case, many kids leave the school premises and pick up lunch at nearby fast food outlets or convenience stores. For them, lunch may be a Slurpee and a candy bar or a monster bag of chips. To all intents and purposes these kids will be brain-dead for the rest of the school day.

Hidden hunger

We think of malnutrition as an issue in underdeveloped countries, but the problem is all around us. Anyone—child or adult—can suffer from what is known as hidden hunger if they subsist on a steady diet of processed foods. This sort of food may satisfy hunger. It certainly contains plenty of calories—far too many, in fact, and way beyond our energy needs. But it does not have enough of the vital vitamins and minerals needed to process those calories and fuel metabolism.

If the word "hunger" conjures up images of thin, frail individuals, think again. Those suffering from hidden hunger today are more likely to be overweight or obese. In North America and throughout the developed world, childhood obesity has reached epidemic proportions and is at an all-time high. In the United States, rates of overweight and obesity have increased two- to threefold over the past twenty-five years. In the United Kingdom, a similar increase has happened more rapidly, in just over ten years.[1] In Canada, rates of overweight and obesity in children aged two to seventeen increased from 15 per cent in 1978 to 26 per cent in 2013. If current trends continue, we should expect to have 70 million overweight or obese children worldwide by 2025.[2]

According to Kul C. Gautam, former deputy executive director of UNICEF, "'Hidden hunger' due to micronutrient deficiency does not produce hunger as we know it. You might not feel it in the belly, but it strikes at the core of your health and vitality." In children, hidden hunger handicaps mental and physical development; in adults, it leads to poor productivity and increases the risk of serious health problems like diabetes and cardiovascular disease.

The causes of hidden hunger are numerous, from poor diet to higher genetic needs for micronutrients in some individuals, to depletion by lifestyle or medications. But whatever the origin of the problem, the solution seems obvious: intervention with supplements to reduce the deficiencies, however caused.

Closing the income gap

Brain imaging shows that the regions of the brain needed for the development of language, reading and executive function tend to be smaller in children from poorer families. As income rises, so does a child's brain size—the cerebral cortex is about 6 per cent larger in children from families with incomes greater than US$150,000 compared to families earning US$25,000 or less.[3]

Intellectual stimulation of young children can help make up for economic disadvantages. Children who grow up in a loving environment surrounded by books and educational toys can achieve optimal cortical development by their late teens, regardless of household income.[4] Creative play boosts the growth of the left temporal cortex, an area of the brain responsible for speech and language recognition, and for semantic memory.

Semantic memory is needed to process the knowledge we acquire over a lifetime. We need it to remember information we are taught—facts or events that are common knowledge, and not acquired through our own personal experience. For example, it is from experience that we learn to avoid touching something that is hot. But we cannot describe the sky on a summer's day unless someone has taught us the word "blue." A well-developed semantic memory is needed to learn to read, to understand mathematics or to remember the capital cities of the world, and is vital for academic success.

Reading to young children, playing with them, and providing toys that teach colours, shapes, numbers and letters helps to develop semantic memory in the early years. In later years, impaired semantic memory may be the earliest sign that dementia is setting in.

Increasing brain demands meet inferior diets

The problem of hidden hunger is even more pronounced in community colleges and universities, where students may be living away from home for the first time. Most don't know how to shop for or cook nutritious food for themselves. Students from poorer homes often have to choose between buying food and paying tuition fees. Fat- and calorie-laden Kraft Dinner, available for pennies at the dollar store, then becomes a staple. Not surprisingly, students commonly gain almost fifteen pounds in their freshman year.[5]

Young women, although more likely to be weight conscious than male students, believe that packing on the pounds at university is inevitable and blame it on their new-found food independence and the influence of friends.[6] While most cafeterias do provide healthy choices, I have watched students on campus walk past the scrambled eggs and grilled tomato on offer for breakfast and instead head straight for boxes of sugary cereal and chocolate milk. They might grab a can of Coke, too. A steady diet of muffins and coffee for breakfast, pizza and Coke for lunch, and a Big Mac for dinner will not only increase the risk for weight gain and diabetes, it's the fast track to malnutrition and an underperforming brain.

Perhaps it's time for college cafeterias not only to offer healthy choices, but to remove the unhealthy ones. The well-being and academic achievement of their students is at stake.

Depression and anxiety growing among teenagers

Psychological distress is rising at an alarming rate among teenagers and young adults. In Ontario, more than a quarter of this age group report psychological distress, and this is higher in female students (36 per cent) than in males (17 per cent). Recent data shows that approximately 15 per cent of teenagers have thought about suicide, although thankfully few of them follow through.[7]

At university, depression and anxiety are the most commonly reported mental health problems, and almost 50 per cent of anxious students said that their anxiety was so intense that they could hardly function.[8] There is a marked overlap between anxiety, depression and drug abuse. Because dopamine naturally suppresses cravings and addictions, low dopamine is thought to be the link between all three conditions.[9]

Dopamine is the great motivator and of all the neurotransmitters, the true antidepressant. It is needed for creative activities; the art student or architectural undergraduate who cannot complete a project may have low brain levels of dopamine. It is needed for articulation and word recall, so the drama or vocal student who can't sustain voice projection or remember lines may well be running short. As we have seen, brain dopamine depends on a meal-by-meal intake of its building block, tyrosine. Protein-rich foods at each meal help keep tyrosine levels high and boost dopamine. Protein in snacks, especially in the afternoon, can be helpful in improving mood and focus.[10]

I find tyrosine supplements are also helpful for students. Even when not anxious or depressed, healthy individuals can benefit from extra tyrosine when under intense mental or emotional pressure.

Dopamine and other nutrients

Of course, tyrosine on its own is insufficient and will not raise brain dopamine levels unless all the other cofactors involved in its synthesis are present. Vitamin C is a prime requirement; after the adrenal glands, the highest concentrations of vitamin C in the human body are found in dopamine neurons. Studies have shown that vitamin C supplements improve mood and decrease anxiety in stressful circumstances. In the 1990s studies showed a direct relationship between IQ and higher serum levels of vitamin C.[11]

Animal studies have found that dopamine is especially sensitive to omega-3 fatty acid and vitamin D deficiencies, both common in student populations. Magnesium is needed to manufacture dopamine and to bind it to adjacent neurons. Classic signs of deficiency are anxiety and depression, and magnesium deficiency is widespread in the student population.

The B vitamins, especially folate and B12, are directly involved in the synthesis of dopamine. However, focusing on only a few of the B vitamins is not helpful. All eight B vitamins have closely interrelated functions, and inadequate levels of *any* of them will interfere with optimal psychological and neurological functioning.[12] Both B vitamins and magnesium are easily depleted by stress.

So in order to maintain high brain dopamine levels, all aspects of nutrition have to be considered together. In Chapter 15 you will find supplement protocols that can be useful for any student overwhelmed by academic life and suffering from anxiety or depression.

ADHD—A growing concern

One of the biggest barriers to learning is attention deficit disorder (ADD) and attention deficit hyperactivity disorder (ADHD). Children with ADHD can't sit still, pay attention or follow instructions. Hidden hunger definitely plays a role: insufficient zinc, iron, magnesium, iodine, vitamin D and DHA in utero and in the first years of life increase the risk of both conditions.[13]

Today, approximately one in ten North American children is diagnosed with either ADD or ADHD—an increase of more than 20 per cent since the early part of the twenty-first century. Some experts think that the numbers are up just because diagnosis has increased, not because the conditions are actually more prevalent. Or, they suggest, ADHD is being over-diagnosed— children who are simply energetic and high-spirited are being labelled with a medical condition. But any seasoned classroom teacher will tell you that the increase is very real. On a daily basis they have to grapple with a grow-ing number of hard-to-manage children in their classrooms.

ADHD runs in families: if a child has been diagnosed with ADHD, at least one parent likely also has the condition.[14] While the symptoms of ADHD may decrease a little with age, they don't necessarily go away. About half the children with ADHD will continue to have symptoms as adults.

Supplements and ADHD

Although ADHD presents challenges in school and at home, good diets and certain supplements can help. Just as we saw for depression and anxiety, dopamine is critical for focus and attention. All the supple-ments that influence brain dopamine levels are also important supports in ADHD. But one additional supplement that has been studied I find particularly helpful.

L-theanine is a unique amino acid found in green and black tea. Experimentally it has been shown to increase alpha brain waves, similar to brain waves produced by meditation. Raising alpha brain waves increases relaxation and a sense of calm. In animal studies, L-theanine increases several neurotransmitters important for learning and memory, including serotonin, dopamine and GABA (gamma-aminobutyric acid).[15] But you would have to drink an awful lot of tea to get the levels necessary to affect brain chemistry.

In Japan, L-theanine has been used for decades as a flavour enhancer and is designated GRAS, as are L-theanine supplements. (GRAS is an acronym for "generally regarded as safe.") One study gave 200 mg of L-theanine, equivalent to twenty cups of green tea, morning and evening to boys with ADHD and found their sleep quality significantly improved.[16] Disturbed sleep is common in ADHD, and the use of stimulant medications to treat ADHD can make this worse.

Because of its relative safety and possible benefits, I use a lot of L-theanine in my practice. I find that both children and adults with ADHD benefit, and I generally recommend 200 to 250 mg of L-theanine on waking and again before tackling homework or assignments. If sleep is a problem, it can be taken again just before bed. Similar doses work for both adults and children.

Diet and ADHD

The Feingold diet is based on a self-help book entitled *Why Your Child Is Hyperactive* published in 1974 by Dr. Ben F. Feingold, MD. In the early 1970s, hyperactivity, as it was then called, was estimated to affect 5 per cent of children. Feingold believed that the artificial food colourings, flavourings and preservatives that had gradually crept into children's diets over previous decades were to blame. He saw tremendous improvements in the behaviour of children with ADHD after they adopted an additive-free diet.

Although some small research studies did show benefit, larger randomized controlled trials did not confirm that there were benefits for the majority of hyperactive children.[17] And so the Feingold diet was dismissed as just another fad diet without scientific foundations— any improvement in children's behaviour was thought to result from attention-seeking children getting special treatment from their parents.

Artificial colourings and preservatives may indeed be a red herring, because excluding foods containing these additives coincidentally cuts out sugar and refined starchy carbohydrates, both of which have neurological consequences.[18] However, many mothers report adverse behavioural reactions in children—even those without ADHD—after exposure to large amounts of synthetic flavourings and colourings. And so the Feingold diet lingers on, but the jury is still out.

Food allergy and behaviour

Another approach sometimes used in ADHD is food allergy testing. Two types of test are used. In a skin prick test, a minute amount of a food is scratched into the top layer of skin. If after fifteen minutes there is a reaction—redness, itching or swelling—the offending food is excluded to see if there are behavioural improvements. Alternatively, a blood test can measure antibodies to a wide variety of foods. High antibody levels are thought to indicate the child is intolerant to that food.

As an immunologist, I'm skeptical about both these tests. Perfectly healthy people can respond to everyday foods like egg, milk and wheat by making antibodies against them, so the tests don't distinguish between those who have a real problem with a food and those who do not.[19] The allergy community acknowledges that both skin prick and blood antibody tests can be wrong as much as 50 per cent of the time—not a solid basis for a lifetime of food avoidance.

While food allergy is a real problem that must be taken very seriously, it affects only a small percentage of the population. Currently the only reliable way to diagnose a food allergy is with an oral food challenge. The suspected food is completely avoided for a period. Later it is reintroduced, and the patient is observed to see if they react. This is the gold standard for food allergy testing, and the only tried and true method of identifying offending foods.[20]

Because of the danger of a life-threatening reaction when the food is reintroduced, this type of avoidance and challenge testing should not be attempted at home and should be done only under the care of an experienced allergist. Lifetime avoidance of any foods identified this way is then necessary.

How to spot an adult with ADHD

Just like children, adults with ADHD have problems with organization. Organizing, as humourist and children's author A.A. Milne put it, is "what you do before you do something, so that when you do it, it is not all mixed up." The lives of adults with ADHD are all mixed up a lot of the time.

Just as the child with ADHD will have difficulty settling down to homework, adults with ADHD procrastinate, putting off essential chores like paying bills or filling out tax forms. They may start a job, break off in the middle and begin something else; halfway through making their bed they might suddenly stop and decide to make a cup of tea. At work, inability to focus and follow through on projects can lead to underperformance and scupper chances of promotion.

Even adults with no formal diagnosis but some of the symptoms of ADHD have impaired quality of life. They are likely to have lower household incomes and a higher rate of unemployment. Because they are prone to impulsiveness, they are often reckless drivers and more likely to speed and have accidents.[21] While many children with ADHD are bouncing off the walls a lot of the time, adults with ADHD are more likely to be edgy and tense, and find it difficult to relax.

What supplements help adult ADHD?

Supplements are important for adults with ADHD. Tyrosine can significantly increase focus and concentration, and reduce procrastination at work and at home. It works well in combination with theanine. L-theanine can help calm the drive to and from work and facilitate relaxation at the end of the day. It is particularly useful to reduce psychological stress in students with ADHD, particularly when academic demands are high.[22]

Like most busy people, adults with ADHD are likely to be short of magnesium, which is both a mental and physical relaxant. One useful way to increase magnesium at the end of the day and to ease tension is to apply a topical form—magnesium gel. Several commercial products are available, or most compounding pharmacies can make it to order in gel or lotion form. Ask for 15 per cent magnesium sulphate or chloride. I suggest avoiding application to any part of the body other than arms or legs—you don't want to apply it too close to sensitive organs like the heart and possibly over-relax it.

Applying magnesium gel to the inner arms or calf muscles (peripheral circulation) gets it into the blood surprisingly quickly. For example, shoulder tension responds within minutes to a good blob of magnesium gel smoothed on the inside of the forearms, where blood vessels near the surface of the skin absorb the magnesium and carry it into the general circulation within minutes. I also suggest that anyone with restless legs or nighttime leg cramps apply it to calves and feet before bed.

Children really benefit from this bedtime routine, especially after they have been involved in strenuous physical activities like hockey or gymnastics earlier in the day.

Choline and ADHD

Choline is the precursor to acetylcholine, also known as the brain's memory manager. Any interference with the production of acetylcholine disrupts memory, focus and attention.[23] Citicoline is a form of choline that occurs naturally in the brain and is also available as a supplement. Under the trade name Cognizin, citicoline has long been used in Europe for the treatment of neurological conditions like Parkinson's disease, and for recovery after a stroke or concussion.

Not only does citicoline increase acetylcholine, it works on dopamine too, stimulating its release from neurons, increasing dopamine receptors, and protecting dopamine-producing neurons from overstimulation, toxicity and cell death. In healthy adults, citicoline can increase focus and improve the retention of new information.[24] While it does not help everyone, I usually suggest a trial of citicoline in adult ADHD, 250–500 mg twice a day.

Researchers gave healthy teenage boys either a placebo, 250 mg or 500 mg of citicoline daily for twenty-eight days and then tested their attention. Compared to placebo, the boys taking citicoline had improved reaction times and reduced impulsivity. Benefits were more pronounced with the higher dose and there were no significant side effects.[25] I find citicoline helpful in teenagers with behavioural disorders. If there is no consistent improvement in memory or attention after three to four months, I usually discontinue use.

Most research on citicoline has been carried out in adults, and its safety and effectiveness in younger children is not known at the time of writing.

Getting the edge at exam time

After they enter high school, the need for children to apply themselves to their studies increases exponentially. For the student with ADHD this is especially challenging. Many will already be taking one of the more commonly prescribed drugs for ADHD, which are stimulants like Ritalin or Adderall. Although it may seem counterintuitive to use stimulants to treat hyperactivity, they work because they increase brain dopamine and norepinephrine, which in turn increases focus and attention. Although effective, these drugs do carry the risk of side effects, some of them serious, like high blood pressure or psychosis.

Prescription stimulant drugs can be abused, moreover. Because they can increase focus and attention, they are commonly sought after by students without ADHD who are cramming for exams.[26] Many legitimate prescriptions for Adderall end up being sold or given away to fellow students.

It isn't necessary to use stimulant drugs illegally to gain the edge in those vital final exams, and the risk of side effects is too great. Severe emotional reactions including hallucinations, panic attacks and psychotic behaviour have been recorded after their use, even when they have been used only briefly. Afterwards, students may feel depressed and lethargic. They may also have extreme difficulty sleeping.

A far better approach—and one that can help students achieve their personal best in exams—is to make sure the brain has all the macro- and micronutrients needed for optimal brain function. Diets should be high in protein to provide the necessary amino acids to manufacture neuro-transmitters like dopamine and noradrenaline. Eggs can provide extra choline needed for acetylcholine synthesis, and fruits and vegetables can provide a sustained-release supply of glucose, the brain's main fuel. This approach not only helps at exam time, but is the cornerstone for lifelong brain health.

In Chapter 14 you'll find the MIND diet described in detail. This is an excellent starting point for students and adults alike looking to naturally enhance cognitive function. The exact protocols for using supplements described in this chapter can be found in Chapter 15.

CHAPTER 12

Into the Workplace

In America . . . when the day's work is done, we go on thinking of losses and gains, we plan for the morrow, we even carry our business cares to bed with us . . . We burn up our energies . . . and either die early, or drop into a lean and mean old age at a time of life which they call a man's prime in Europe . . . What a robust people, what a nation of thinkers we might be, if we would only lay ourselves on the shelf occasionally, and renew our edges!

MARK TWAIN,
The Innocents Abroad

After the relaxed atmosphere of school and college, the workplace can be daunting. Never mind having to learn new skills; just figuring out how fit in in a new and unfamiliar environment can keep you awake at night. For the seasoned worker, a new position is just as stressful. This next step up the ladder may be what you've wanted, but once in the job you may be plagued with worries and uncertainty. Will you be an effective leader and meet the demands of the job? If you have been promoted within the same workplace, will former co-workers accept you as their new boss?

Some jobs are inherently stressful. First responders like firefighters, police officers and soldiers live with unavoidable and unpredictable daily stress. But any job will be stressful if there is constant conflict. Workplace stress can create a daily burden that is harmful to health. Whatever the source of stress, implementing the dietary and supplement advice in Chapter 6 can be immensely helpful.

Fuelling the brain at work and at play

Most people think of food as fuel; if we get hungry, we know we need to eat. But if we think of food simply as fuel, then we probably also feel that anything that satisfies that hunger will do. So we grab a doughnut and coffee, or some pot noodles. If we have to attend an important lunchtime meeting where no food is served, a candy bar may have to do. Oh well, you think. I'll have a proper meal for dinner tonight. But what happened the last time you did that? How well did you work in the afternoon? Just like kids at school, adults at work need to sustain their brains with the right nutrition.

And it's at work that we give our brains the toughest workout. When neurons fire in a particular area, the blood capillaries expand in that region to deliver extra glucose and nutrients. When we are reading, for example, the occipital cortex—the region at the back of the brain that processes visual information—is highly active. When we are challenging our brain mathematically, perhaps working on a spreadsheet, then neurons are firing in the intraparietal sulcus, located toward the top and back of the brain.

Our ability to do these tasks will be excellent when our blood is rich in oxygen and essential nutrients. But when concentrations are low, we may struggle.

Hard-working brains need more B vitamins

Earlier I discussed a study where researchers gave healthy young adults either a placebo, multivitamins containing just the recommended daily intake (RDI) of B vitamins, or ones containing three times the RDI. When these subjects were asked to perform difficult mental tasks, those given the higher levels of B vitamins had significantly improved cerebral blood flow. Not only did the high-dose group perform better on memory and other cognitive tasks, their physical stamina improved.[1]

And both groups performed better than the group given a placebo. As the authors of that study commented, "If it is possible to beneficially modulate core physiological processes such as energy metabolism and cerebral blood flow by simply administering vitamins and other micronutrients to healthy members of the population, then *it must be the case that the nutritional status of the sample, and by implication, the general population is inadequate"* (my emphasis).

From diet alone it would be difficult to get the high levels of B vitamins used in this study, which suggests that supplementing with B vitamins is necessary if hard-at-work brains are to function as well as they could.

Of mice, men and gorillas: More about vitamin C

As we saw in Chapter 6, animals like mice, rats, cats and dogs manu-facture their own vitamin C from glucose, which we cannot do. The adrenal glands have first call on our vitamin C, and animals that can make vitamin C immediately ratchet up their production when they are stressed. Primates like chimpanzees, gorillas and humans that cannot synthesize vitamin C depend on diet to provide enough.

The gorillas of the Congo eat a largely vegetarian diet. Throughout the day they eat continuously, grazing on leaves, bark, stems, roots, vines, bamboo, wild cherry, thistles and nettles—fresh vegetation that is rich in vitamin C.[2] A gorilla weighing 180 kg (400 lb.) eats 30–35 kg (65–75 lb.) of vitamin-C-rich foods in a day.[3] While it's hard to get exact data on the vitamin C content of the forest plants gorillas eat, 30 kg of spinach, for example, would contain approximately 8.5 g of vitamin C. Gorillas spend 60 to 70 per cent of their waking days foraging, so their continuous intake of vitamin-C-rich foods mimics the continuous pro-duction of vitamin C by animals that synthesize it.

Of course the average male gorilla weighs much more than the aver-age human. But if vitamin C requirements were similar for us, a 90 kg (200 lb.) man would need to consume around 4 g of vitamin C daily, and a 68 kg (150 lb.) woman about 3 g—equivalent to 10–15 kg of spin-ach. Adults consuming the bare minimum five servings of fruits and vegetables a day, according to our healthy eating guidelines, will get about 200 mg of vitamin C—more than enough to satisfy current RDIs for vitamin C (75 mg for women; 90 mg for men). While this intake will prevent scurvy, it beggars belief that this is sufficient to cover our increased needs during periods of illness or stress. Certainly no studies have systematically looked at the vitamin C needs of stressed humans.

If you take a vitamin C supplement, make sure it is time-released—that is, formulated to continuously release small doses of vitamin C over ten to twelve hours. This also mimics the eating patterns of primates in the wild.

What happens when you feed gorillas the wrong diet?

What happens when we remove gorillas from their natural habitat and keep them in zoos? Are they as healthy as if they were roaming wild? Do they live as long? It seems not. Gorillas in captivity die prematurely. Just like humans they are overweight, and just like humans they frequently die from heart disease.

At the Cleveland Zoo in the United States they took a long hard look at how they fed their gorillas, and they didn't like what they saw. Daily rations were a bucketful of vitamin-rich, highly processed food, loaded with fat, starch and sugar—the common gorilla fodder used by most zoos. So the Cleveland Zoo changed the gorillas' diet to one more closely reflecting that of their brothers and sisters in the wild.[4]

Now, every day each gorilla receives a wheelbarrow full of greens and fibre-rich foods—romaine lettuce, dandelion greens, endive, alfalfa, green beans and flaxseed, as well as young tree branches from which the gorillas strip and eat the bark and leaves with relish. Hidden inside a banana, they get three human multivitamin and mineral pills. All the food is hidden or strewn around the animal enclosure so that the gorillas are constantly on the move foraging for their new diet.

The results have been astonishing. Although the new diet provides many more calories than the old one, the gorillas are losing weight, as well as total body fat. The researchers plan to investigate changes in markers for heart disease and diabetes, like cholesterol, glucose and insulin levels in their blood, hoping that the new diet has a positive effect on heart disease and longevity.

"We're beginning to understand we may have a lot of overweight gorillas," said Kristen Lukas, an adjunct assistant professor of biology at Case Western Reserve University and chair of the Gorilla Species Survival Plan for the Association of Zoos. "And, we're just recognizing that surviving on a diet and being healthy on a diet are different. We've raised our standards and are asking, are they in the best condition to not only survive but to thrive?"[5]

Are modern diets at odds with evolutionary diets?

If only we were as thoughtful about human diets as the zookeepers at the Cleveland Zoo are about gorilla diets. Current daily recommendations for most essential nutrients are focused simply on survival. But that's no longer enough. We want to thrive, not just survive. We want to avoid or postpone for as long as possible the onset of the chronic diseases that compromise our ability to enjoy a long and active life, like heart disease, diabetes, hearing and vision loss and, of course, dementia.

How closely do we resemble our great ape cousins? Genetic research has shown that humans, chimps and gorillas evolved from a common ancestor about 10 million years ago. Chris Tyler-Smith, a geneticist at the Wellcome Trust in the United Kingdom, says, "The big picture is that we're perhaps 98 per cent identical in our [genetic] sequences to gorillas. So that means most of our genes are very similar, or even identical to, the gorilla version of the same gene." That includes genetic needs for vitamin C.

The paleolithic or paleo diet is an attempt to mimic human hunter-gatherer diets, aligning today's dietary intake with the sort of foods that would have been available to our early ancestors. Those who adhere to this style of eating consume mainly meat, fish, eggs, fruits and vegetables, nuts and seeds, as well as healthy fats like olive and coconut oil. They avoid all dairy, cereal products like bread and pasta, and legumes like lentils and beans. Although there are several versions of the paleo diet, one feature is common to them all: heavily processed food is avoided. A growing body of evidence supports the idea that the processing of modern food is harmful, producing diets that are nutritionally inferior—loaded with calories, sugar and fat, and low in protein, fibre, vitamins and minerals.[6]

Research consistently shows that compared with the standard fare consumed by the average North American today, a paleo diet can reduce the incidence of heart disease, control weight and prevent the onset of dementia.[7] But while I think that many of the paleo diet recommendations make a lot of sense, such an approach to eating may be unnecessarily restrictive. An alternative is to focus on eating whole, minimally processed foods, as outlined in Chapter 14.

The problem with processing

The most important dietary shift at Cleveland Zoo is that the gorillas are no longer fed highly processed foods. Instead their food is unprocessed, meaning it's jam-packed with fibre and health-enhancing phytochemicals, and low in added sugar. The animals are also supplemented with daily multivitamins and minerals. Some scientists are calling for a similar shift in human diets.

Dr. Jean-Claude Moubarac, PhD, a Montreal-based medical anthropologist and specialist in public health, thinks many of our current health problems are rooted in our high consumption of ultra-processed foods. These foods may have started life in a field, river or cow barn. But en route to our bellies they passed through factories where they were depleted of nutrients and fibre, and made palatable by the addition of sugar, salt, and chemical colourings, flavourings, thickeners, emulsifiers and preservatives.

These ready-to-eat, ready-to-heat foods are made from cheap, nutritionally bankrupt ingredients and are high in calories. Ultra-processed food contributes 90 per cent of added sugar to American diets.[8] In Canada, a Senate committee report on obesity highlights the fact that Canada's Food Guide is dominated by ultra-processed foods—a factor that must shoulder some of the blame for the obesity epidemic.[9] This change from home-cooked, unprocessed or minimally processed foods to ultra-processed, ready-to-consume foods has been the biggest change in our eating patterns in the last hundred years.

As diets have shifted to ultra-processed foods, so have waistbands expanded. As the Senate committee stated, "There is an obesity crisis in this country and Canadians are paying for it with their wallets and with their lives."

Performance anxiety and busy brains

For some people, standing up to make a speech or giving a presentation to a group of colleagues creates serious stress. Others may dread face-to-face meetings with colleagues or customers. Any work situation where you have to be articulate and focused will drain brain dopamine and affect performance. Imagine going into your boss's office to ask for a raise. Your heart is beating out of your chest, your palms are sweaty and you're terrified you'll forget all your carefully marshalled arguments about why you deserve this raise. You are now short of dopamine.

Without sufficient dopamine, a lawyer might have difficulty putting together a cogent argument in court. A teacher might be hesitant or get confused when explaining new concepts to students. Concert pianists or opera singers might suffer from stage fright and fail to deliver their best performance. If we chronically lose focus or concentration when we are put in stressful situations, we can develop serious performance anxiety. And that may mean resorting to medication just to function.

But there is a solution to performance anxiety: tyrosine supplements can enable us to replace dopamine and make up for losses caused by stress.

Do healthy people benefit from tyrosine?

Sylvia was a high-flying scientist, well-known on the international conference circuit. A slow convert to using supplements, she believed that her excellent diet would supply her with all the nutrition she needed. Gradually, though, she began to feel that supplements might be helpful. "I take my supplements regularly," she told me. "Even if I just end up peeing them out, I still think they are a good insurance policy."

I hear that argument often: supplements just make expensive urine. Certainly you do find extra vitamins and minerals in the urine of those who take supplements. But does that mean we got no benefit from them as they passed through? You might just as well argue that we're better off not drinking water. After all, we only pee it out—why waste time on trips to the bathroom? But water is important to hydrate and detoxify tissues. We'd laugh if someone told us drinking water was a waste of time because eventually we would just pee it out.

One evening I was having dinner with Sylvia. She had been reading about tyrosine in a previous book I wrote. "I can't believe what a difference it makes to take tyrosine just before I have to speak," she said. "The words just flow." Sylvia is one of the smartest, most articulate and confident people I know. For me her comment was a clear example of how stress—even the stress we seem to handle with ease—can limit dopamine production. If Sylvia felt a difference when she took tyrosine, then probably anyone in stressful situations can benefit from boosting dopamine production through tyrosine supplementation.

The busy brain syndrome

You know the feeling: thoughts race round and round in your head—the work you didn't complete at the office, the list of things the kids need for their school trip tomorrow, the argument with a colleague or family member. This busy brain syndrome is a prime reason we can't relax at the end of the day. In healthy individuals, L-theanine can dampen down this sort of brain overactivity and stop the constant chatter in our heads.[10] It's not just for those with ADHD.

The busy brain can stop us sleeping. Alpha brain waves are needed to create the right conditions for sleep. Meditation—letting go of random thoughts and blocking intentional thinking—is one way of inducing alpha brain waves. Fine, if you are a practised meditator. But if you are not, taking L-theanine before bed can have a similar effect.

As we have seen, sleep is not an optional extra. Without sleep, we cannot clear the brain of the accumulated garbage generated during the day—the brain's glymphatic system is simply non-functional. During the night we also set the hormones that will control the next day's appetite and metabolism. If we do not sleep, then appetite increases and we can consume an extra three hundred calories. Women are especially inclined when sleep deprived to choose high-fat, high-calorie junk foods, like ice cream. If we are prone to weight gain, chronic insomnia can sabotage our ability to control food intake.

Circadian misalignment

Even if we sleep reasonably well but are night owls—staying up very late at night and sleeping later in the morning—we are likely to eat later and continue snacking on the wrong foods at night. This is called circadian misalignment. Circadian rhythms are changes in physical, hormonal and behavioural responses that occur roughly every twenty-four hours, and are linked to phases of light and darkness.

Circadian misalignment and disturbed eating patterns not only lead to obesity but also increase the risk of heart disease, diabetes and cancer. Short sleeping also increases the risk of depression, attention deficit disorders and even schizophrenia. It is common in patients with mild cognitive impairment, and may be a sign that MCI will later progress to Alzheimer's disease.[11]

Many clients I see intentionally cut short their sleep. They may work late at the office and feel the need for some downtime when they get home, so they delay going to bed. But then they get up early to go to the gym before work, and in total sleep barely five hours a night. In my practice I work hard to optimize sleep for all clients, not just those with chronic insomnia. I also try to get people to change their sleeping practices and get to bed earlier.

A night owl myself, I have started to put my alarm on, not just to wake me in the morning, but also to remind me when it's time to go to bed. Try it—it works.

Serotonin and dopamine—Balance and synergy

Several neurotransmitters, including acetylcholine, noradrenaline, GABA (gamma-aminobutyric acid) and histamine are involved in regulating the sleep-wake cycle, but the two most studied are dopamine and serotonin. They are also two neurotransmitters that are relatively easy to manipulate with nutritional supplements. As we have seen, for focus and concentration we need dopamine to dominate during the working day. Taking tyrosine supplements on waking, and perhaps again during the middle of the afternoon, will maintain dopamine levels during the working day.

When the day's work is done, it's time for serotonin to take centre stage. Dopamine is stimulating, allowing information to access the brain. Serotonin does the opposite: it screens out sensory information and is calming. The precursor molecule or building block for serotonin is the amino acid tryptophan. Unlike tyrosine, which becomes essential only under conditions of stress, tryptophan is always essential.

While tryptophan is present in protein foods, overall its concentration is low. Because of this, tryptophan has difficulty crossing the blood-brain barrier, being elbowed out of the way by other, more plentiful amino acids. When we eat a small sweet snack, though, something magic happens: blood sugar rises, followed closely by an increase in circulating insulin. Insulin binds most amino acids and takes them off to muscle cells for repair and maintenance. But it doesn't bind tryptophan. Now, with all the competition out of the way, tryptophan easily crosses the blood-brain barrier and brain serotonin rises. This is one reason we call foods that quickly and easily raise insulin levels "comfort foods."

Many people overeat heavily processed carbohydrates like potato chips or cookies when they are stressed. These foods certainly make us feel better temporarily. But they won't help us work efficiently, because afterwards we'll feel drowsy and unfocused. We're also likely to gain weight. This trick of nature—the urge to eat sugar or carbs when worried or stressed—is common in women suffering from premenstrual syndrome.

It is also common in anyone attempting to give up smoking. Nicotine increases serotonin secretion, and nicotine withdrawal reduces brain levels, so a recovering smoker may instinctively turn to other ways to raise brain serotonin.[12] No wonder many people who quit smoking gain weight rapidly in the following year.

Birds do it, bees do it

Sleep-like states probably occur in all animals—elephants, birds, reptiles, even insects. In humans, more than eleven days without sleep is fatal. We can't survive without it. Although scientists don't yet understand *why* we need to sleep, it is clear that we must. Sleep deprivation lowers our mood and our cognitive and physical performance.[13]

The sleep-wake cycle has three main phases: we are either awake, in slow-wave sleep or in rapid eye movement (REM) sleep. Once the brain is awake, it uses dopamine to maintain itself in this state. Gradually over the course of the day serotonin builds up in the brain, and eventually sufficient serotonin accumulates to trigger the onset of sleep. We then enter the first phase of sleep, slow-wave or deep sleep. Muscles relax. Heart rate, blood pressure and body temperature fall. Growth hormone, needed for cell and tissue repair and replacement, is released. During slow-wave sleep, memories are transferred from short-term to long-term storage.[14] Deep sleep is therefore both physically and mentally restorative.

After a period in slow-wave sleep we enter REM sleep, also called paradoxical sleep. Apart from the muscles of our heart and lungs, the rest of our body is paralyzed. This is when active dreaming takes place, signalled by the rapid movement of our eyes backward and forward under closed eyelids. Blood pressure, heart rate and breathing are very variable during REM sleep.

REM sleep stimulates parts of the brain needed for learning, which may explain why infants spend so much time in REM sleep. REM sleep is important for our emotional well-being. When we are deprived of it, our emotional reactivity may be higher the next day. Over time, prolonged disruption of REM sleep leads to increases in anxiety and depression.[15] Slow-wave and REM sleep cycles are repeated several times during the night, with the slow-wave sleep becoming less deep and the REM periods more prolonged as the night goes on.

Sleep remedies from the health food store

If we can influence dopamine levels during the day by taking tyrosine, can we influence nighttime serotonin levels using supplements? Tryptophan itself is sometimes used as a sleep aid. While it works for some people, it's not the most efficient route to increasing brain serotonin, since only about 1 per cent of tryptophan consumed gets into the brain. Another reason tryptophan may be less effective is that if niacin (vitamin B3) is in short supply, we will use tryptophan to make it. This depletes tryptophan, leaving little left to manufacture serotonin. Tryptophan can also be sidelined for the biosynthesis of other structural body proteins.

Once in the brain, tryptophan is converted to 5-hydroxytryptophan (5-HTP), which in turn is converted to serotonin. 5-HTP is available as a supplement, derived from the seeds of an African plant called *Griffonia simplicifolia*. Approximately 70 per cent of supplemental 5-HTP gets into the brain, and I find it more effective than tryptophan for sleep. The dose needed is highly individual, so start with 100 mg just before bed. If that works, fine. If not, gradually increase the dose in 50 mg increments up to 300 mg.

If you tend to wake after three or four hours of sleep, I recommend leaving 50–100 mg beside the bed with a glass of water and taking it when you wake.

Melatonin—The darkness hormone

Ultimately serotonin must be converted to melatonin, sometimes called the darkness hormone. Melatonin is made in the pineal gland, a pea-sized gland located in the centre of the brain. Melatonin is needed to regulate circadian rhythms—how well we sleep tomorrow night depends on whether we manufacture enough melatonin tonight.

Provided we have sufficient serotonin at the end of the day, we should be able to make our own melatonin. But beware. We can only manufacture melatonin when we are asleep in the pitch dark. Even tiny traces of light—streetlights coming around the edges of the bedroom curtains or a hall light showing under the door—will prevent melatonin's manufacture. If you cannot create complete blackout in your bedroom, it's wise to wear an eye mask.

Even in large doses melatonin is relatively nontoxic, but as with 5-HTP it's best to take only just enough to help you sleep. Start with 3 mg, taken sixty to ninety minutes before bed. Gradually increase until you find the dose that will make you sleepy at your desired bedtime. Plan to be ready to go to bed an hour or so after you've taken melatonin—don't fall asleep in an armchair watching TV. If you do, you will wake up some time later having missed the critical window of opportunity for sleep induction and may not sleep when you do get into bed.

Why not use one of the many over-the-counter or prescription sleeping pills available? Many sleeping pills alter normal EEG patterns and the ratio of REM to non-REM sleep. Melatonin and 5-HTP, however, are natural to the body. They are the biochemical materials that the brain normally manufactures to put itself to sleep. Taken correctly, 5-HTP and melatonin can help us fall asleep and stay asleep, without disrupting normal sleep rhythms.

5-HTP may be ineffective if the many vitamins and minerals needed to manufacture serotonin and melatonin are missing. Magnesium is particularly important, and people who optimize their magnesium intake as outlined at the end of this book often find a significant improvement in sleep quality and quantity. Nighttime leg cramps, restless leg syndrome and waking frequently to pee are signs of low tissue stores of magnesium.

Other important nutrients involved in melatonin production include B vitamins, vitamin C, iron and zinc. These can be provided by a daily multivitamin and mineral supplement.

Brain busters in the medicine cabinet

"I guess it's just my age" or "I'm having a senior moment" are common ways of explaining away early signs of memory loss. In my office such excuses are discouraged: we know memory loss isn't an inevitable consequence of aging. One culprit for deteriorating cognitive function, pharmaceutical drugs, may be hiding in the bathroom.

Drugs called benzodiazepines (such as Valium and Ativan) are frequently prescribed for anxiety or insomnia. The benzodiazepines work by interfering with the transfer of memories from short-term to long-term storage. While this might be desirable in the short term when under extreme stress, in the long term these drugs can lead to permanent memory loss, especially in those who are carriers of the ApoE4 gene—a gene that influences our ability to regulate cholesterol metabolism and increases the risk of dementia.[16] Most knowledgeable pharmacists recommend that benzodiazepines be used only for brief periods.

In fact, all the drugs used as sleeping aids obstruct the normal transfer of new memories into long-term storage. In the short term these drugs may dampen anxiety and help you sleep, but the price you pay may be a gradual decline in your ability to learn and remember new material. In computer terms, the data fails to get saved to the hard drive.

Of course, sudden withdrawal of drugs is never advisable and can sometimes cause disturbing side effects, so you should only ever stop medications on the advice of a physician.

Drugs linked to increased risk of dementia

Many prescription and over-the-counter drugs can raise the risk of cognitive decline. In particular, the proton pump inhibitors (PPIs) used to treat indigestion and reflux significantly increase the risk of dementia.[17] PPIs are frequently overprescribed—by some estimates up to 70 per cent of prescriptions are unnecessary. As we have seen, these drugs seriously deplete magnesium, which is essential for the production and function of neurotransmitters. They also inhibit the absorption of B12 and increase the risk of B12-deficiency dementia.

The blood thinner warfarin has been in use for more than half a century; an estimated 20 million Americans take this drug for atrial fibrillation, an irregular, quivering heartbeat. Long-term users of warfarin for this purpose increase their risk of dementia.[18] Other common drugs that have been shown to increase dementia risk include antidepressants, drugs prescribed for bladder control and antihistamines.[19]

This area of research is a fast-moving field, with new associations between drugs and dementia being uncovered all the time. Ask your pharmacist if there are risks associated with any medications you may be taking.

Statins, cholesterol and cloudy thinking

Early animal studies suggested that increased levels of cholesterol promoted the production of amyloid and "cloudy thinking."[20] So it seemed reasonable to see whether statins—drugs that block the manufacture of cholesterol—might also prevent Alzheimer's disease. However, there is growing concern that far from protecting the brain, these drugs actually may increase cloudy thinking.

Kenneth was a fifty-eight-year-old man, the husband of a client of mine. Sitting in my office, he described a recent experience that puzzled and concerned him. A week earlier he had met an old workmate he hadn't seen for some time and they had dinner together. After an enjoyable evening they parted company but by coincidence bumped into each other the following morning. Kenneth had no recollection of meeting his friend. In fact, he couldn't even remember having dinner at all. He had experienced a condition called transient global amnesia.

Kenneth had recently started to take a statin drug to lower his cholesterol. He wondered if there was any connection between his memory lapse and starting this new drug. Searching the Internet he found an alert from the U.S. Food and Drug Administration acknowledging that, although rare, forgetfulness and confusion could occur in statin users. Problems usually cleared up several weeks after stopping the medications.[21] Kenneth stopped taking the drug and had no further episodes.

Statins have become the darlings of the medical profession. There have even been suggestions that, regardless of cholesterol levels, everyone over forty-four should be taking them.[22] But these drugs cross the blood-brain barrier and interfere with cholesterol production. As we saw in Chapter 5, cholesterol is vital to brain functioning, so it's not unreasonable to think that statin drugs could affect brain health negatively. And most individuals can effectively treat high cholesterol through lifestyle and dietary changes, so why take the chance?

CHAPTER 13

What to Do If Memory Fails

Memory is all we are. Moments and feelings, captured in
amber, strung on filaments of reason. Take a man's memories
and you take all of him. Chip away a memory at a time and
you destroy him as surely as if you hammered nail after nail
through his skull.

MARK LAWRENCE,
King of Thorns

Suppose in middle age we begin to experience symptoms of serious memory loss: Must we resign ourselves to an inevitable and progressive decline? Should we prepare ourselves and our family for the worst? Or can we take steps that could delay further memory deterioration, or even reverse it?

Early diagnosis is crucial

Kate Swaffer is a dementia patient with an inspiring personal story.[1] At the age of forty-nine, she was diagnosed with early-onset semantic frontal lobe dementia. As we have seen, we use semantic memory to recall information we learned when we were children. Semantic memory has been compared to a mental combination of dictionary and encyclopedia, with a thesaurus thrown in for good measure. We need it to know the word "apple," be able to spell it, pronounce it and describe it. Semantic memory also links the word "apple" to descriptive words like "round," "juicy," "small," "edible," "grows on trees." But if semantic memory starts to fail, we may be unable to find the word for "apple," and instead say "cherry."

Kate was devastated by her diagnosis. She was advised to go home, give up her job and get her affairs in order. It was suggested that she attend a daycare for Alzheimer's patients at least once a month to "get used to the idea" and prepare for the inevitable. Kate had imagined her fifties quite differently. She had planned to go back to college and pick up the studies she had abandoned years ago. But the doctors insisted these were dreams she would have to give up.

Kate almost accepted the doctors' advice. But something inside her resisted being written off so easily. Not willing to let go of her dreams, she sought advice and support from organizations that help people overcome other types of learning problems and doggedly pursued her university courses. She earned two undergraduate degrees and continued on to study for a doctorate. She became an activist and spokesperson for Alzheimer's Australia.

What is clear from Kate's experience is that, if diagnosed early enough, patients with dementia can and do go on to lead happy and productive lives, albeit with certain limitations. As with any handicap, a new way of learning and living is needed. Twenty years ago, doctors and nurses were seeing only patients in the later stage of the disease. But today, patients like Kate are being diagnosed earlier, at a point when there are still unexplored possibilities for rehabilitation.

Early diagnosis is critical, and finding ways of diagnosing the disease in its early stages is a major research focus. But what is disappointing is the lack of information on the potential for nutritional support in the rehabilitation process.

Depression and nutrition

Celeste first came to see me many years ago when a physician friend recommended that she seek nutritional help for the chronic depression she had suffered from all her adult life. She had tried medication without much success—the drugs made her feel sleepy constantly. She lost her appetite but at the same time began to put on weight. Celeste might have accepted these side effects had the antidepressants not made her feel unbearably anxious. She stopped taking them.

One thing that did help was exercise. Every day she played long and exhausting games of doubles tennis, after which she felt tired but relaxed and, temporarily, almost euphoric. "It's the only way I can cope," she told me. But the benefit didn't last long, and by the next day her mood was low again. She found it difficult to take pleasure in anything. No matter how happy people were around her, her mood never changed—it always seemed flat.

Celeste was a teacher, recently retired. She had two adult children, one of whom had been born with spina bifida. Hearing this immediately rang alarm bells for me, since one common link between depression in a mother and spina bifida in her baby could be unmet needs for folic acid. Folic acid is needed for the manufacture of serotonin, and deficiency is a known risk factor for depression.[2] Celeste was aware of the relationship between folate deficiency and spina bifida, but not of its association with depression.

Seeing the daily struggles of her handicapped daughter was a major source of Celeste's stress and depression. "I would willingly have taken folic acid when I was pregnant," she told me despondently, "but nobody told me I needed to."

Just one deficiency, or many?

Of course, folate is just one of the nutrients that can lead to depression when in short supply. Others include omega-3 fats, vitamin D, other B vitamins, vitamin C, magnesium and zinc. For at least two of these— vitamin D and omega-3 fats—widespread deficiencies exist in the general population, and these deficiencies can compromise the ability to make and use serotonin.[3]

Celeste had no real interest in food and ate only when she thought about it. I encouraged her to eat three meals a day, to include lots of vegetables and fruit, and to make sure she had protein at each meal, not just dinner. I explained that since depression was linked to so many nutrient deficiencies I would want to work on a comprehensive supplement regime for her. To fix one apparent deficiency without considering the likelihood of others would be a wasted effort; like mending just one hole of many in the bottom of a leaky boat, it wouldn't keep the boat afloat.

Celeste started on a multivitamin, daily fish oil, extra vitamins C and D, and magnesium. Because some individuals have genetic difficulties processing folate into its active form, methyltetrahydrofolate, I added a separate supplement containing this form of folate. I suggested tyrosine supplements to deal with the ongoing stress in her life. I also suggested she modify her exercise regime to one that was less physically stressful, but she was not prepared to do this—tennis was not only psychologically important to her, it was the focus of her social life.

Because magnesium is so important for brain health and magnesium supplements have been shown to reverse depression,[4] I made sure she optimized her magnesium intake. Even if she didn't have special needs, her extreme physical activity coupled with stress was a daily drain on her magnesium. Within a few months Celeste was feeling considerably better. She reported better mood, more energy and less irritability. She even felt her tennis game was improving.

Supplements help only if you take them

For several years Celeste came back to see me regularly, but I can't say she was ever really consistent with her new diet or supplement regime. She'd be compliant for a while and then fall off the wagon. Even though she admitted that she felt worse when she wasn't eating properly or taking her supplements, she was still inconsistent. After some years she stopped coming to see me altogether.

One evening I was giving a lecture at a local church hall when I spotted her in the audience. She lived locally and had seen the announcement of my talk in the church bulletin. During a break for refreshments she came up to talk to me. "I have some bad news," she whispered. "I've just been diagnosed with frontal lobe dementia. Can I come back and see you?" It was seven years since we last had spoken.

In my office I could see that this well-educated and formerly articulate woman was having difficulty communicating. She was still the same intelligent person I had known, but now her speech was slow and hesitant. She stuttered frequently and complained that she couldn't "get the right word out." Sometimes she used wrong or unrelated words, or mispronounced them. She explained that she had had to learn to simplify what she wanted to say. "I can only use little words now," she said.

Her behaviour had changed too. She was more anxious and restless. She told me that her irritability now frequently turned into aggression. Her depression was so profound that at times she felt suicidal. She still played tennis, but her stamina was poor, and her serves and volleys were getting more and more erratic. A long-time bridge player, she had given up her usual Thursday evening game with friends because she simply couldn't remember what cards had been played.

A dreaded diagnosis

Celeste had initially gone to see a neurologist at one of the country's top neuroscience centres after she began experiencing mood changes and speech problems serious enough to be noticed by her family. At the clinic she was put through a battery of cognitive tests and had a CT (computerized tomography) scan of her brain, which can help distinguish between true dementia and simple depression. The scan showed atrophy in the frontal lobes.

Another type of scan—a SPECT (single photon-emission CT) scan—was also done. By measuring blood flow, a SPECT scan measures brain activity. In Celeste's case the SPECT scan confirmed that blood flow and therefore activity in the frontal lobes appeared to be nonexistent. On the basis of brain imaging studies and a battery of other tests, Celeste was diagnosed with the semantic variant of frontal lobe dementia.

The frontal lobes contain most of the dopamine-sensitive neurons in the cerebral cortex. Remember that dopamine is not only a major mood booster; it is also critical for articulation and word recall. And because dopamine is consumed when we make adrenal hormones, stress dramatically depletes it. As we have seen in past chapters, taking tyrosine—the amino acid used to make dopamine—can boost brain dopamine and offset stress-related dopamine depletion.

Celeste had stopped taking tyrosine supplements, although she had previously found them helpful in treating her depression. She had also dropped her intake of vitamin D, even though past testing suggested she needed a higher than average daily dose to maintain good blood levels. Vitamin D activates the genes that release dopamine and serotonin from neurons, and even mild vitamin D deficiency doubles the risk of dementia and Alzheimer's disease.[5] She had continued taking the special folate supplements I had earlier suggested.

She had also continued to take B12 but at a lower dose than before. On testing, her blood level was low at 178 pmol/L. Although this level is within the reference range quoted by the testing laboratory, and therefore considered normal, blood levels under 300 pmol/L have recently been shown to be linked to generalized brain shrinkage in older individuals.[6] And just as in pregnancy, the ratio of folate to B12 is important. Low B12 coupled with high blood folate—common in countries like Canada where food is fortified with folic acid—increases the risk of memory problems.[7]

Celeste went back on all the supplements I had originally recommended for her depression. But with this new diagnosis I thought we should consider two additional supplements.

Choline and memory

We have seen how choline is critically important during pregnancy, altering brain structure in the developing baby. A high intake of choline by the mother influences lifelong memory in her offspring.[8] We can make a little choline ourselves, in the liver. Premenopausal women are a little better at doing this than men, probably because of the extra need for choline during pregnancy. But deprived of choline, both men and women develop fatty livers and muscle damage.[9]

Drugs that recycle acetylcholine, called cholinesterase inhibitors, stop acetylcholine breakdown, and while they may not cure dementia or stop its progression, they can help lessen some of the symptoms, at least for a limited time. So cholinesterase inhibitor drugs like Aricept are often the first treatments tried in early-stage dementia. However, people with frontotemporal dementia don't usually do well on these drugs, and may even become more agitated.

I encouraged Celeste to eat at least one egg a day and take a choline supplement to raise brain acetylcholine without drugs. I suggested she take the same form of choline—citicoline—that had shown benefit in attention deficit hyperactivity disorder, discussed in Chapter 11. Citicoline, also known under the trade name Cognizin, has shown some benefit after traumatic brain injuries and strokes, and in patients with vascular dementia and Parkinson's disease.[10] In healthy middle-aged women citicoline supplements can improve attention and focus.[11] But choline supplements are not a panacea: the results of several recent large randomized clinical trials of citicoline in stroke and traumatic brain injury patients have been disappointing.

Why clinical trials of nutrients so often fail

Large randomized clinical trials (RCTs) are the mainstay of pharmaceutical research. In an RCT, people are randomly assigned to take either a drug or a "sugar pill" (placebo) to see whether the drug is better than taking nothing at all. Occasionally the drug may be compared to an older drug to see if it is an improvement over what is already on the market.

RCTs are the gold standard for testing the efficacy of drugs. But they are unsuitable for testing multiple different combinations of compounds that may interact, like vitamins and minerals. Apart from being prohibitively costly, any such trial would have to include enormous numbers of patients and would take too long to be practical.

One group of researchers tried to estimate how long it would take to test the seven possible treatments for Alzheimer's disease. As we have seen, no single drug has proven effective in Alzheimer's disease, but the researchers thought that combining several different drugs targeting different neurological pathways might be more effective. The researchers calculated they would have to complete 127 separate RCTs, enrolling 63,500 patients. Moreover, the project would take 286 years to complete.[12] Now imagine the difficulty of studying forty different nutrients in various combinations. It would be quite impossible.

There are also ethical factors to consider when studying vitamins that don't apply to drugs. In a drug trial you can be certain that the placebo group is not taking the study drug, so it's a clear-cut comparison between the treatment group and the control group. But because vitamins are essential for life itself, you cannot deplete the control group without harming them. And vitamins are present to a greater or lesser extent in food, so depending on their diet the control group is always consuming an unpredictable amount of the vitamin being tested. The distinction between the treatment and control group is therefore not clear-cut.

Unfortunately, scientists test essential nutrients as if they were drugs without recognizing that you simply cannot get reliable data by studying vitamins one at a time. All the essential nutrients are required to maintain and repair the brain and regulate the innumerable processes required for memory and brain function. Deficiency of any one therefore affects brain health.

To quote Jeffrey Blumberg of Tufts University, one of the most influential voices in nutrition research, "We have this really complicated issue, because there are so many different nutrients which play important roles in promoting health and in preventing the diseases we are looking at. So, to do a simple study of [for example] just vitamin E and heart disease isn't so simple when you recognize that you need to control for all these other nutrients."

The problem with studying complex systems

Suppose the auto industry makes the claim that properly adjusted spark plugs are essential for cars: that without them cars will not start, and if they are not properly adjusted, the car will not run well. Although common sense might suggest that the car manufacturers are right, how can we test this assertion?

If we followed the current logic of vitamin research, we would obtain a number of cars that were not working, put in new spark plugs and see if we could get the cars to start. One or two cars might. But when a significant number of cars failed to respond, we wouldn't be entitled to conclude that spark plugs are useless. If we did, we might expect to draw a scathing response from the auto industry and leave knowledgeable car owners shaking their heads in disbelief.

But this is exactly what we do with vitamin research. We test vitamins in isolation, and when we can't get them to work on their own, we discard them as useless or possibly even harmful. While the scientific approach that reduces everything to studying one variable at a time may work for drugs or for surgical interventions, it is doomed to fail when we try to study complex systems. Some thoughtful researchers are at last beginning to see the limitation of this approach and have called for a moratorium on vitamin research until we can figure out how to study nutrition in all its complexity.[13]

In the meantime, we should remain skeptical about negative or confusing results from clinical trials that focus only on one essential nutrient, ignoring all the others it interacts with.

Vitamin E and the brain

Another supplement I thought Celeste should take was the fat-soluble antioxidant vitamin E, which helps to protect the brain's white matter. Following a stroke, vitamin E has been shown to prevent the development of white matter lesions.[14]

When we take supplements of any nutrient we are basically enhancing the nutritional content of our food. Supplements should therefore mimic as closely as possible the nutrients present in food. Some supplements are the same (bioidentical) whether they are synthetic or from food. Vitamin C is a good example: the body cannot distinguish between synthetic vitamin C and the vitamin C in an orange. Synthetic vitamin E is another matter. In nature, vitamin E exists in eight different forms: four of them are classified chemically as tocopherols (alpha, beta, gamma and delta) and four as tocotrienols (again, alpha, beta, gamma and delta). As antioxidants, the eight forms all do something slightly different but work synergistically and so should be taken together.

Dl-alpha-tocopherol is a synthetic version of one of the eight forms of vitamin E. High doses have been shown to slow the progression of Alzheimer's disease when given together with cholinesterase inhibitors.[15] But this form of vitamin E is unlikely to have the same advantages as full-spectrum versions. In fact, it may even do harm, since excess dl-alpha-tocopherol can block absorption of other beneficial forms of vitamin E from food.[16]

One study in Finnish individuals eighty years and older showed that those with highest blood levels of *all* forms of vitamin E had a lower risk of cognitive impairment, with each of the eight forms playing a unique role.[17] Unfortunately, for too long the medical and scientific communities have assumed that alpha-tocopherol was the only form of vitamin E worth studying. Moreover, many studies have used the cheap and readily available synthetic version—dl-alpha-tocopherol—which is not identical to natural alpha-tocopherol.

So great is the ignorance around the different forms of vitamin E that many studies don't even bother to mention which form they use, a fact rarely picked up on by the journals that publish their research.[18] This omission makes it impossible for other researchers to accurately reproduce the original studies and contributes to growing confusion in the research literature.

Needless to say, I suggested the full-spectrum form of vitamin E for Celeste. And, despite negative medical reviews, I suggested she start taking 250 mg of citicoline twice a day.

I get it, I finally get it!

Celeste continued in the dementia program. She worked with a speech pathologist to improve her verbal fluency. The therapist would show her pictures and ask her to name the items in them. At home she had to practise naming colours and shapes every day, which she did faithfully. She continued taking her supplements, this time more consistently.

It was harder for her to adjust to the dietary guidelines. These were the same guidelines I had suggested years ago but which she had never really taken seriously. She was not used to eating regularly and often skipped meals. She also found it hard to consume the ten daily servings of vegetables and fruit that offer the greatest health benefit. But now she worked on optimizing her diet. Out with the sugar and processed starchy foods; in with the protein, vegetables and fruit. One day I received an email from her with the subject line "I get it, I finally get it!"

She had begun to see how much better she felt when she ate properly and remembered to take her supplements.

After a year the consultant neurologist commented that Celeste was doing better than had been predicted when she was originally seen. "For someone with your diagnosis, you are certainly high functioning," she commented. Some months later the consultant told Celeste she could see no reason for her to continue in the dementia program: they could no longer find evidence of the memory and language problems she had presented with two years earlier. In fact, they were sure she did not have frontal lobe dementia. Leaving the doctor's office, Celeste sat in her car and wept.

Celeste asked the doctor what might have caused the problems that brought her to the clinic in the first place. "Well," the neurologist replied. "You were under a lot of stress. That probably caused your symptoms." The doctor was right, of course. Prolonged and intense stress can damage the brain and, as we have seen, one mechanism for this damage may be the depletion by stress of the nutrients required for brain function. Celeste's lifelong battle with depression suggested that her brain had higher nutrient needs than most.

I believe that it was because she began to satisfy those needs that Celeste began to recover. And she thought so, too.

What to do if memory starts to fail

Get enough sleep. Only when we sleep can the brain remove the cellular debris that has accumulated during the day. Melatonin can help regulate sleep. It is also a powerful antioxidant that can protect the brain from damaging free radicals. One study gave 3 mg of melatonin to Alzheimer's patients for four weeks. Both cognition and sleep improved.[19]

Most people need seven to eight hours of sleep. Sleep in a pitch-dark room, or wear an eye mask. To personalize supplements for sleep according to your needs, follow the instructions in Chapter 12.

Exercise. Exercise increases blood flow to the brain and helps generate new blood vessels. It also stimulates the birth of new neurons in the hippocampus, promotes brain plasticity and increases cognition.[20] As a minimum, take a brisk walk for thirty minutes, three or four times a week.

Adopt a brain-friendly diet. Heart-friendly diets like the Mediterranean diet and the DASH (dietary approaches to stop hypertension) diet are also brain friendly. The MIND diet outlined in Chapter 14 is a hybrid of these two, and seems more effective than either one, reducing the risk of Alzheimer's disease by 53 per cent when followed faithfully.[21]

Eat lots of colourful vegetables and fruit. Convincing evidence shows that inadequate intake of vegetables and fruit is at the root of many of today's health problems, including dementia. Diets that are veggie-centric (not necessarily vegetarian) contain an array of phytochemicals that are antioxidant, detoxifying and anti-inflammatory.

Although five-a-day might be what many dietary guidelines recommend, in the case of vegetables and fruit, more *is* better. Aim for the ten daily servings that have been shown to confer the best health. Herbs and spices are rich sources of phytochemicals and can add health to a meal without adding calories. Wherever possible, enrich meals with these chemical powerhouses.

Start a basic supplement regime. If you are not already taking supplements, begin the basic regime outlined in Chapter 15. Your program should include a multivitamin and mineral complex, fish oil, extra vitamins C and E, and magnesium. Vitamin D and magnesium should be optimized to your own personal needs (see Chapter 15).

Add memory-targeted supplements. If memory problems persist, try adding extra L-tyrosine, L-theanine and citicoline to your basic regime. Add them one at a time, leaving several weeks in between, to see which ones are beneficial.

Ideally, work with a knowledgeable practitioner who can help you build a program of memory-supporting supplements that is optimal for you.

Get tested for vitamin D. Without a blood test you can't tell if you are deficient in vitamin D. Try taking 4,000 IU (100 mg)—the upper limit of vitamin D and the amount anyone from the age of nine onward can take without supervision or fear of adverse effects. Test your blood level after three months. However, if the end of your three-month trial falls in the summer months, wait until November to test. If your results are in the top end of the normal range by then, fine. If not, work with a knowledgeable practitioner to find out how much vitamin D you should take to correct this.

Check vitamin B12. Vitamin B12 is needed to preserve the myelin sheath around the neurons and to manufacture neurotransmitters. If you have a blood test for B12, don't accept reassurances that you are "normal" just because you are in the laboratory reference range.

In my practice I suggest keeping B12 levels high—between 1,000 and 2,000 pmol/L (1,350–2,710 pg/mL)—to balance the high blood folate values that are almost universal since food fortification. B12 in this range has been linked to improved energy and well-being.[22] You will need to take a B12 supplement (as methylcobalamin, the active form) to achieve these levels.

I recommend taking 1 mg of methylcobalamin daily and then rechecking B12 in three months. Because no side effects have been reported from high blood levels of B12, there is no official upper limit to the amount you can safely take.

Optimize magnesium intake. Low dietary intake of magnesium may contribute to cognitive impairment and needs to be corrected. Especially if you are constipated, you're going to need more magnesium than is usually present in a multivitamin. Follow the instructions in Chapter 15 to adjust your magnesium intake to your bowel tolerance.

Not only will this relieve constipation, it may prevent the progression of memory loss.[23]

Learn to relax. Relaxation can positively influence brain chemistry by shutting down the release of brain-damaging stress chemicals into the bloodstream. Learn to meditate or use other well-researched relaxation practices.

Progressive muscle relaxation is a technique in which muscles are repeatedly tensed and then relaxed. It is easy to learn—you can teach yourself using one of the many instructional videos on the Internet. Progressive muscle relaxation can calm an overactive brain[24] and help with stress and anxiety. It also helps with insomnia.

A new day dawns

At the Alzheimer's Research Center at UCLA, Dr. Dale Bredesen, MD, is taking a new approach to studying early-stage dementia: investigating multiple factors that can potentially increase the risk of Alzheimer's disease, including thirty-six nutrient deficiencies and imbalances, lack of exercise, excess stress and insufficient sleep.

In a small preliminary study, nine out of the ten patients saw a reversal of their symptoms within three to six months. Six patients in the study had stopped working or were struggling with work when they joined, and all were able to improve their performance and return to work. The one patient who did not improve had late-stage Alzheimer's disease.[25]

"The existing Alzheimer's drugs affect a single target, but Alzheimer's disease is more complex. Imagine having a roof with 36 holes in it, and your drug patched one hole very well. The drug may have worked, and a single hole may have been fixed, but you still have 35 other leaks, and so the underlying process may not be affected much," Bredesen commented.[26]

Although these results need to be confirmed in larger studies, I believe the outcome is pointing the way to a more successful approach in early-stage dementia, one that will involve a combination of interventions. No single approach, one drug or individual nutrient will be the solution. The main lesson to be learned from Celeste's case is to try multiple different dietary approaches. And not to give up.

PART 5

Planning Strategies

CHAPTER 14

Shopping Smarts: Budget-Conscious Choices at the Grocery Store

To eat is a necessity, but to eat intelligently is an art.

FRANÇOIS DE LA ROCHEFOUCAULD

Over the course of evolution, populations in different parts of the world have survived on a variety of diets, with local variations in climate and geography dictating what food was available. Because of brutally high infant mortality rates, overall life expectancy was not high for our hunter-gatherer ancestors. Surprisingly, however, if they made it past the age of fifteen, their life expectancy was very similar to ours today.[1] The fact that early populations survived on many different combinations of foods suggests that a wide variety of eating patterns provided enough energy and sufficient essential nutrients to support growth to maturity and reproduction. But even for those who did survive into middle age, it is unlikely that their diets provided sufficient nutrition for *optimal* health.

Today, as the miracles of modern medicine extend our lifespan further and further, our desire is not just to live a long life, but to make those extra years as disease-free as possible. Current research suggests that if we are to protect our hearts and minds from premature deterioration and live healthy long lives, our diets must improve.

Protective, less protective and non-protective foods

As we saw in Chapter 4, the earliest worldwide effort to provide guidance on how to eat for health was developed by the League of Nations after World War One and first published in 1935. Under that scheme, food was divided into three groups: highly protective, less protective and non-protective. People were told to focus their eating mainly on food in the first group, eat some (but not a lot) of the less protective foods and avoid non-protective foods.

Highly protective foods included fish, vegetables and fruit, milk, cheese, butter and eggs. For full health, a weekly serving of liver was considered necessary to provide extra iron. And a daily serving of cod liver oil, by that time known to prevent rickets and other diseases caused by vitamin D deficiency, was also recommended. (Incidentally, cod liver oil also provided more omega-3 fats, although these were not yet on the nutritional radar screen.) The importance of protein was stressed, and 1 g per kilogram of body weight was recommended for all adults, with more for pregnant and nursing women. This is above today's standard recommendations in North America, which consider 0.8 g of protein per kilogram body weight to suffice. As we have seen, research suggests that even this is not optimal and 1.2 g is more realistic.

Less protective foods included meat, starchy vegetables like potatoes and turnips, as well as legumes like dried peas and lentils. Cereal-based foods like rice, pasta and bread were also in this group, and no distinction was made between white and wholewheat bread or white and brown rice. The non-protective foods included sugar, jams and jellies, and honey. Where possible these were to be avoided, since they provided lots of calories with little or no nutrition. The concept of nutritional density was stressed. Nutritionally dense foods give you the most nutrients for the least amount of calories.

Unprocessed, minimally processed and ultra-processed food

Today, instead of our diets being based on nutrient-dense foods, in most wealthy countries they are top-heavy with *energy*-dense, ultra-processed foods: bread, cookies, cakes, fries and snack foods like chips and sodas. These provide many more calories than we need but little nutrition.

The *British Medical Journal* defines ultra-processed food as "industrial formulations which, besides salt, sugar, oils and fats, include substances not used in culinary preparations, in particular concepts used to imitate sensorial qualities of minimally processed foods."[2] In other words, they look like food and taste like food but are really chemical concoctions designed to trick our taste buds. Between 1938 and 2011 the most important change in Canadian dietary patterns has been the replacing of unprocessed or minimally processed foods with ready-to-consume, ultra-processed food products.[3]

The great food writer Michael Pollan has a more user-friendly way of describing ultra-processed foods: "edible food-like substances." I love that expression. It perfectly describes foods like hot dogs, pizza pockets, breakfast cereals, packaged bread products, processed cold cuts, ready to heat and eat frozen entrées, cookies, chips and many other packaged foods that make up the bulk of groceries in many shopping carts.

Pollan suggests that to avoid ultra-processed foods we should not buy any food that is advertised on TV. We should read food labels and shun any product that contains more than five ingredients. And if there are chemical names on the label that a seven-year-old can't pronounce, give that food a wide berth.

Processed foods are cheaper

But the fact remains that processed foods, with their added sugars, hydrogenated fats, flavour enhancers, emulsifiers, artificial sweeteners and preservatives, are inexpensive and convenient. They also have the highest profit margin for manufacturers.

Nutritionist and economist Barry Popkin at the University of North Carolina, commenting on how cheap packaged macaroni and cheese is compared to fresh fruit and vegetables, says, "We have a processed package food industry which is enormously efficient. It takes a little bit of wheat. It takes a little bit of artificial cheese. It uses lots of chemical flavors and it makes these magical tasty foods that are very inexpensive."[4] By contrast, more nutrient-dense foods like lean meats, fish, fresh vegetables and fruit generally cost more.

In Canada, 60 per cent of the food we consume is ultra-processed, and the proportion is similar in the United States.[5] The sad truth is that for decades governments have subsidized the raw ingredients used in the manufacture of fast food. Even though they advise us to severely limit our intake of these foods, they are the foods our governments help to make cheap.

According to Popkin, "We didn't really create the same infrastructure for fruits and vegetables that we created for animal foods, for oils, sugars and other things. The difference is such a huge magnitude of long-term investment that it would take an awful lot to make fruits and vegetables cheap like they should be."

And if you think eating according to Canada's Food Guide will help, think again. Despite pretty good adherence to our government-sanctioned guidelines, Canadians are getting fatter and sicker. As we saw earlier, a damning report was issued by a Senate committee looking at the root causes of Canada's growing obesity epidemic. It heavily criticized Canada's Food Guide as "at best ineffective, and at worst, enabling" the growing obesity crisis and the rise in chronic degenerative diseases like diabetes, heart disease, cancer and dementia. The most likely reason for the failure of Canada's Food Guide is that it allows too many ultra-processed foods. In fact, you could easily comply with its guidelines while eating mostly ultra-processed "edible food-like substances."

Getting value for money

So how can we get the healthiest foods without breaking the bank? Most of the cost of ultra-processed food represents processing, transportation and advertising. For example, 2006 data from the Food Marketing Institute shows that the cost of marketing foods consumed in the United States accounted for 81 per cent of the total cost to the consumer. Only 19 per cent of the purchase price went to the farmers.[6] As Pollan says, we need to stay away from foods that are heavily advertised. Where possible, avoid packaged food, which is usually the most processed. This is often referred to as "shopping around the edges of the supermarket," where the fresh produce is usually stocked, and avoiding the central aisles where most of the packaged foods are displayed.

To get the best value for money, stick to seasonal vegetables and fruits. These can be very cost effective. And if you buy them at a farmers' market, you know you are putting money straight into the farmer's pocket—the transportation and packaging costs are minimal, and advertising costs are zero.

Start to cook more meals at home. It can be fun to learn just how much money you are saving by making a quiche or meatballs yourself. A U.S. study found that those who spend more time in the kitchen preparing family meals are more likely to eat a healthy diet and have a significantly higher intake of vegetables, salads and fruit. They also spend less on food, saving on average seven dollars per family member per week.[7]

Does healthy food cost more?

Despite evidence to the contrary, the perception persists that if we want healthier food we have to spend more money. While foods like organic free-range eggs or milk or beef from grass-fed cows may indeed be pricier than their factory-farmed equivalents, we are easily tricked into paying more than we should for many foods if we believe they are healthier for us.

A team of researchers at Ohio State University designed a series of experiments to test whether the price alone of a food could affect our perception of its health value. Test subjects were presented with a new product labelled the "Healthiest Protein Bar on the Planet." Half the participants were told the bar would retail at $0.99 and the other half were told it would cost $4.00. Then they were all given the opportunity to read reviews of the product before giving their own opinions. Those told the bar would cost $0.99 scoured the reviews carefully, unable to believe that something so cheap could be any good. But the group that thought the bar cost $4.00 were much less likely to read the reviews, taking it on faith that something that cost twice as much as the average protein bar was bound to be healthier.

In another experiment, participants were asked to imagine that a colleague had asked them to pick up lunch for them. Half the group were told that their co-worker wanted something healthy, while the other half got no specific instructions. Given two options to choose from that were identical in nutritional content—either a roasted chicken wrap priced at $8.95 or a "Chicken Balsamic Wrap" for $6.95—people invariably chose the more expensive roasted chicken over the balsamic chicken wrap. But when the prices were reversed, so were their choices. Participants had assumed that the more expensive the wrap, the healthier it had to be.[8]

The lesson from this research is that to eat well on a limited budget, we have to become discriminating shoppers. Price is not always the best guide to quality.

The MIND diet

Heart-friendly diets like the DASH (dietary approaches to stop hypertension) diet and the Mediterranean diet have both been shown to be protective of brain health and can help slow memory loss as we age.[9] The DASH diet, promoted to prevent high blood pressure and other risk factors for heart disease, focuses on reducing sodium while eating healthily. The Mediterranean diet is the traditional diet of Greece, southern France and parts of Italy. Both diets are based on a high intake of fruits and vegetables, lean meats, fish, nuts and beans, grains, olive oil and grilled or steamed chicken and seafood. The Mediterranean diet also allows a daily glass or two of wine.

A hybrid of both diets, the MIND diet (Mediterranean-DASH intervention for neurodegenerative delay) is an attempt to take common elements from the DASH and Mediterranean diets that are thought to confer the most health benefits, and create an eating pattern that is tasty, supports brain health and is easy to follow. Certainly the MIND diet is easy to remember: it consists of only fifteen foods, ten of them healthy and five unhealthy. Even if you don't follow it exactly, research suggests you can still reduce your risk of Alzheimer's by 35 per cent.[10]

Although the MIND diet looks simple, its recommendations are a little more complex to implement than they appear at first sight.

Ten foods to eat

1. Green leafy vegetables: one salad a day
2. Other vegetables: one serving a day
3. Nuts: one serving a day
4. Berries: two or more servings a week, blueberries and strawberries preferred
5. Beans: three to four servings a week
6. Whole grains: three servings a day
7. Fish: one or more servings a week
8. Poultry: at least two servings a week
9. Olive oil: this should be your primary oil
10. Wine: one glass a day

Five foods to avoid

1. Red meats: eat rarely
2. Butter: eat no more than a tablespoon a day; never eat margarine
3. Cheese: one serving or less a week
4. Pastries and sweets: avoid all
5. Fried or fast food: less than one serving a week

Is MIND really the best we can do?

While the MIND diet is certainly a great deal better than the average North American diet—sometimes referred to as the SAD (standard American) diet—I am not sure that it is optimal for brain health. For example, hard-working brains can benefit from higher intakes of phytochemicals than provided by the daily serving of leafy greens and one other vegetable and the twice-a-week serving of berries in the MIND diet. And the MIND diet does not take into account the processing of food. Whole grains that are pulverized have a high glycemic load, just like refined grains. The MIND diet does not distinguish between beneficial foods in their natural state and those that have been changed by processing.

Butter, as we have seen, is not as dangerous a food as we have been led to believe. Of course the quality of the butter matters—it should be made from organic milk from grass-fed animals. Apart from being lower in added herbicides and pesticides, organic milk has a better nutritional profile. It is higher in omega-3 fatty acids and vitamin E compared with conventional cow's milk.[11] And the research on red meat is confusing since so many studies have included heavily processed meats like sausages and luncheon meats under the umbrella term "red meat." While these should be avoided, a small grass-fed steak now and then may be a different matter.

Nutritional research has a tendency to conclude that because something is shown to be "better" for us, it is necessarily the best we can do. While the MIND diet is an excellent place to start your healthy eating journey and is relatively simple to follow, it can certainly be improved on. I believe that you can significantly enhance it by incorporating some—preferably all—of the rules below.

Seven science-based rules for brain-healthy eating

1. Eat mainly unprocessed foods. Unprocessed foods are as close to their natural form as possible. They include fish, poultry, eggs, milk, nuts and seeds, fresh or frozen fruits and vegetables, and fresh and dried herbs and spices. Minimally processed foods are also part of a healthy diet but should be eaten in smaller quantities. They include olive, coconut or flaxseed oil; canned beans or lentils; yogurt, butter and cheese; nut butters like almond or peanut butter; and nut milks.

Cooking itself *is* a form of processing, but it is acceptable, and can make food more digestible and, in some cases, more nutritious. Many phytochemicals are better absorbed from cooked foods. For example, lycopene, one of the red-yellow-coloured phytochemicals, is better absorbed from cooked tomatoes than from raw. Lycopene is important for brain health and plays a role in preventing prostate cancer. On the other hand, phytochemicals present in cruciferous vegetables, which include broccoli, cauliflower, collard greens and kale, also have important cancer-fighting properties, but these are generally reduced by cooking. Eating these vegetables raw or lightly steamed is therefore best.

Although many phytochemicals have been studied in the laboratory, many more have not. There are probably countless substances with substantial health-giving properties that we have not yet discovered, let alone knowing whether they are better eaten raw or cooked. Personally, I hedge my bets by eating a range of both raw and cooked vegetables daily.

2. Eat nutrient-dense food. These are foods that give you the most amount of nutrition with the fewest calories. An egg is a perfect example: at only about 70 calories, a large egg contains 7 g of protein and many vitamins and minerals, including brain-friendly choline. Egg whites provide low-calorie protein, but it's the yolks that contain the choline and most of the vitamins and minerals. Four or more eggs a week can prevent the development of type 2 diabetes.[12] Eggs also appear to reduce the risk of certain cancers and improve cognitive function with age. And despite what we have been taught, we do not need to worry about increasing heart disease risk if we indulge in eggs. Up to one egg a day has no impact on stroke or heart attack risk, even in those already experiencing heart failure.[13] Where possible, choose eggs that are free range and organic.

Fruits and vegetables are also nutrient dense, and most are low in calories. Nuts, seeds and butters made from them contain plenty of fibre, phytochemicals and good fats. Nuts make a convenient snack and have proven benefits for heart health. But a little goes a long way—they are also high in calories. Limit yourself to about one-third of a cup daily.

3. Bump up your intake of vegetables and fruit. This means focusing daily menus on vegetables and fruit for a "veggie-centric" diet, although not necessarily vegetarian. Don't forget, fruits and vegetables are carbohydrates and are the brain's most nutritious source of essential glucose. While it is true that grain-based carbohydrates like bread, pasta, rice and potatoes also provide the brain with glucose, depending on how processed they are and how they are cooked, they have a higher glycemic index (see rule #4 below). Eaten regularly throughout the day, fruits and vegetables more efficiently provide the steady supply of fuel our brains need to function efficiently, as well as an array of health-giving phytochemicals. These protective molecules help to shield the brain from inflammation and defend it from free radical damage. While free radicals are damaging to any organ or tissue, the brain is particularly vulnerable to this type of damage.

So gradually increase your daily vegetable and fruit intake until it is optimal—ten servings a day for adults and an age-appropriate number for children, as outlined in Chapter 7. Vegetables should dominate: aim for a balance of seven vegetables to three fruits. Limit the sweeter fruits like banana and pineapple to occasional treats. Instead, choose less-sweet fruits like blueberries, apples and under-ripe pears. For weight control choose above-ground vegetables like leafy greens, fresh or frozen peas and beans, broccoli and cauliflower, tomatoes, cucumbers, zucchini, peppers and other salad stuff. Remember you need a little fat to absorb phytochemicals, so always eat fruits and vegetables with something that contains fat. Even when you are working hard to increase your total servings, you can still deprive yourself of their full benefits if you eat them without fat.

To achieve that magic number of ten daily servings, you need to include either vegetables or fruit or both with every meal or snack. For breakfast, for example, shun the temptation of a fruit-bottomed yogurt with all its added sugar. Instead, have a bowl of mixed berries topped with plain yogurt or cottage cheese and a sprinkling of nuts or granola. When you have more time at the weekend, have an omelette with mixed grilled vegetables—red and green peppers, onions, and mushrooms. Having boiled or scrambled eggs for breakfast? Add a fresh tomato.

Take cut-up raw vegetables to work and snack on them with some hummus or tzatziki, a low-calorie yogurt-based dip. Or slice up an apple or pear and spread the slices with a little almond butter or cream cheese. Lunch could be leftover stir-fried vegetables from last evening's supper or a mixed salad. Add some cold chicken and an olive oil–based salad dressing for a well-rounded midday meal. Start dinner with another salad and serve at least two vegetables with the main course. A bowl of berries can be up to two servings (1 cup) and makes the perfect dessert. Before long you will be surprised at how many servings you can cram into your day.

4. Eat a low glycemic load. Limit yourself to one serving of starchy food per meal. If you eat bread, make it as unprocessed as possible. Eliminate breakfast cereals and white flour–based products. Root vegetables like potatoes, sweet potatoes, parsnips and beets can be healthful but can have a high glycemic index. They should be limited to one serving per meal and should be used to replace other high-glycemic foods like bread, pasta and rice. If hungry, fill up on extra vegetables rather than bread. The following are serving sizes of starchy carbohydrates:

1 slice of wholegrain bread
½ cup cooked brown rice
½ cup cooked wholegrain pasta
¼ wholegrain bagel

When eating out, beware of the warm bread rolls that arrive at your table almost as soon as you've taken your seat. Watching other diners eat can make us hungry and impatient for our own food to arrive. So this restaurant ploy fills us up at the start of a meal and keeps us busy while we wait for our own food to be prepared. But far from filling you up, bread may leave you feeling hungrier than before because its high glycemic index will trigger a spike in insulin. Dealing with the crash in blood sugar that follows may be why we reach for a second or even third roll. Try asking for a plate of olives to nibble on instead. Or sip a glass of sparkling water with a slice of lemon in it, and take a pass on the pre-dinner bread ritual.

Avoid fruit juices. Although they do contain plenty of those good phytochemicals, they also contain too much sugar. An orange contains about three to four teaspoons of sugar and, eaten whole, this sugar is slowly absorbed. But a glass of orange juice is another matter, since an eight-ounce glass contains the sugar of three oranges—ten to twelve teaspoons. And because the fibre has been removed or pulverized, blood sugar spikes rapidly after we drink it.

5. Remember that fat is not optional. Good fats are essential for healthy brains. The list of good fats below includes many that we may have unfortunately learned to avoid during the low-fat craze. Include them freely in your everyday diet for increased health and vitality.

avocado
seafood, such as shrimp
fatty fish (salmon, trout, herring, sardines)
nuts, especially walnuts and almonds
nut butters, such as almond and peanut butter
olive oil
coconut oil
eggs, yolks included

Include olive oil in your salad dressing. At snack time have a small piece of cheese or some yogurt with your fruit. Have a knob of butter on your broccoli or spinach without guilt—the vegetables taste so much better, and the fat helps you absorb their valuable phytochemicals and fat-soluble vitamins like A, D, E and K.

6. *Watch protein intake.* Despite repeated claims that North Americans eat too much protein and fears that excess protein might cause bone loss and kidney damage, research has found that we actually don't get enough, especially if we are pregnant, very physically active or over the age of sixty-five. Spreading protein out over the day is the healthiest way to consume it. Most of us need 25–30 g of protein with each meal, which translates into the following:

3–4 oz. of chicken, turkey or other meat
⅔ can of tuna
8 medium shrimp
1 cup of cottage cheese
2½ cups of Greek yogurt
3 cups of regular yogurt
4 eggs
1½ cups of lentils
3 cups of cooked quinoa

1¼ cups of tofu

7 tablespoons of peanut butter, or 100 almonds

Remember that our bodies cannot store excess protein for future use and we should therefore eat only as much protein as we can metabolize at any one meal. Excess will be turned into fat—a process that is hard on the liver and kidneys. You will notice from the above list that meat, poultry and fish provide high-quality protein with the fewest calories; they are nutritionally dense foods. To get enough protein from quinoa at one meal you would have to eat an excessive amount of starch.

7. Practise mindful eating. In North America, we eat too fast. It takes at least twenty minutes from the time we start eating for our brains to register our food intake, and therefore tell us whether or not we have eaten enough. Eating slowly allows us to digest our food properly as we eat, while speed-eating not only interferes with digestion but results in overeating. Many studies link eating too fast with weight gain.[14] So slow down and enjoy every mouthful. Take small bites of food and chew it well. If necessary, watch the clock so you spend at least twenty to thirty minutes eating a meal.

Even if all the foods we consume over the course of a day are healthy foods, too much of a good thing can still be a bad thing. A Japanese proverb cautions that "eight parts of a full stomach sustain the man; the other two sustain the doctor." People in Okinawa, Japan, live by this maxim, and Okinawans are some of the healthiest, longest-living individuals in the world. Many are living a full and active life at one hundred years of age. So try to finish a meal and leave the table when you are about 80 per cent full. In the long run it will pay off with better heart health and a trimmer waistline.

Mindful eating also means cutting back on food waste. We cannot complain about food bills if a significant amount of what we buy ends up in the garbage. In the United States, approximately 25 per cent of food purchased gets tossed out by the end of the week, costing an average family of four an estimated US$1,365 to US$2,275 annually.[15] Wasted food also has a negative effect on the environment, since it decomposes in landfills to produce methane, a potent greenhouse gas that contributes to global warming. Before you go shopping, check to see what's already in the refrigerator that needs using up before it goes bad.

An assortment of leftover vegetables can be quickly transformed into a tasty stir-fry with the addition of some protein—perhaps chicken breast, or some fresh or tinned salmon. A favourite Saturday lunchtime meal for me is what my family called "end of the week soup." A lonely carrot, a few stalks of celery and a potato, all roughly chopped and sautéed in olive oil, are then simmered with some herbs and spices in beef or vegetable broth. A cup of red lentils makes this a thicker, more substantial soup, and leftover cooked chicken or beef makes it a complete meal. For colour I add some frozen peas or green beans when it is almost cooked. A handful of arugula, kale or spinach added at the end also provides nutrition and colour.

In my kitchen, the tough outside leaves of lettuce not pretty enough to be used in a salad are tossed in a bag in the freezer and later added to smoothies. This way I can easily add another serving of vegetables without many calories. You can also wash the skins of lemons, oranges and clementines before you peel or squeeze them, and then save them in a bag in the freezer. Citrus peel added to smoothies not only enriches with extra health-giving phytochemicals but also provides a delicious burst of flavour. Why throw away the stalks of cauliflower or broccoli and use only the florets? The stalks are just as tasty and nutritious. Grated or finely shredded, they can have a new life as coleslaw or in stir-fries.

Many useful websites feature ways to combine the leftover food sitting in your refrigerator into a quick and easy meal. Just key the word "recipe" into your favourite search engine followed by the ingredients you want to use. Any number of tasty suggestions will pop up. And don't sweat the small stuff. Ignore the hype around the latest "superfoods" and just get used to eating regular meals of good wholesome foods, and eating them in their natural form, as unprocessed as possible. Don't worry if you are not always able to afford organic food—you still need to eat your fruits and vegetables. Finally, enjoy your food and the time you spend preparing it. Your health depends on it!

CHAPTER 15

Supplement Protocols

Vitamins are like seat belts. Wearing a seat belt doesn't give you a license to drive recklessly. It just protects you in case of an accident.

JEFFREY BLUMBERG, PhD

General advice on taking vitamin and mineral supplements

While supplements can never replace a healthy diet, many of us still benefit from additional micronutrients, even when we eat very carefully. On the flip side, no amount of supplements can compensate for careless eating. This is because food contains many other valuable nutrients, such as fibre and phytochemicals, that confer major health benefits. There may even be elements in foodstuffs important for health that we have yet to identify.

As we have seen, our needs for the essential nutrients vary depending on our age, our sex, our size and also our current state of health. Many of the medications used to treat common health conditions also deplete vital vitamins and minerals that, if not replaced, could lead to new, possibly more serious, health conditions. For example, the class of drugs called proton pump inhibitors, such as Nexium and Losec, deplete magnesium and as a consequence may increase the risk of heart attacks.[1]

An additional twist to the whole conundrum of whether it is wise to take vitamin and mineral supplements is the recent science confirming the long-held belief that we are all biochemically unique and that our personal genetics also influences our needs. Daily requirements can vary between individuals anywhere from threefold for thiamine (B1) to forty-fold for iron. While current recommended daily intakes provide the minimum needed for survival, they cannot possibly be optimal for everyone.

Despite the wide disparities in individual needs, some general guidelines can help us when choosing supplements. There are also some nutrients we can, with a little effort, personalize to our own specific requirements, such as magnesium and vitamin D.

Selecting a multivitamin

If you take nothing else on a daily basis, a multivitamin should be your first choice. A good multivitamin contains a little bit of most vitamins and minerals and can be a useful insurance policy against nutritional gaps. Remember, no nutrient works alone. Each one depends on a host of other nutrients to work effectively and efficiently.

While there are good multivitamins intended for use by both men and women, it's generally best to choose a brand that makes different male and female versions, and formulates them for different age groups. For example, men over fifty and postmenopausal women are likely to have slightly different needs compared to their younger counterparts. Choose a product that contains the widest spectrum of trace minerals—the trace mineral molybdenum is a good indicator of completeness. It should also contain 15–30 mg of zinc. Don't worry if your multivitamin contains relatively low levels of magnesium, since it is too bulky to include in a multivitamin at the levels that you probably need. Similarly, vitamin C is rarely present in sufficient amounts. You will need to supplement both these nutrients separately.

As we've seen, the brain's need for B vitamins probably far exceeds the recommended daily intakes, especially if we exercise vigorously or work our brains hard. Start by choosing a multivitamin that contains at least 25 mg of most of the B vitamins and 400 µg of folic acid. For optimal brain health, take a separate B12 supplement. As we have seen, a balance of folic acid and B12 is important for brain health, and although multivitamins contain ample folic acid, it is rare to find one that contains sufficient B12. I recommend an additional 1 mg daily of the activated form of B12, methylcobalamin, either in drop form or as sublingual lozenges. This is the form that is best absorbed and retained in the body.

Vitamin C

The upper limit of vitamin C is 2 g a day for adults. I generally suggest 1 g of vitamin C twice a day (1 g = 1,000 mg). Remember that the definition of "upper limit" is the amount anyone in a specific age group can consistently take, without supervision and with minimal chances of side effects. The table below shows the upper tolerable limit for all age groups.

Children			Teens	Adults
1–3 years	4–8 years	9–13 years	14–18 years	19 years and older
400 mg	650 mg	1,200 mg	1,800 mg	2,000 mg

Our cousins the great apes graze on vitamin-C-rich foods all day long. This continuous intake of vitamin C throughout the day may in part compensate for losing the ability to make vitamin C on demand, as is the norm in the rest of the animal kingdom. We can mimic the gorilla's continuous foraging if we take time-released vitamin C, formulated to gradually release vitamin C into the circulation over ten to twelve hours. I recommend this form of vitamin C, since most other forms are rapidly lost from the body.

Vitamin D

Living in northerly countries—forty degrees latitude or higher—during the winter months puts everyone at risk of vitamin D deficiency. In these regions vitamin D deficiency is especially common in the elderly but can also affect younger age groups, particularly anyone who is housebound, wears sunblock or covers up extensively while outdoors.

Compared with light-skinned people, those with dark skin need much longer exposure to sunlight to make equivalent amounts of vitamin D and are therefore particularly at risk of health problems associated with vitamin D deficiency. This is especially true for those who move from sun-rich regions like the Caribbean or Central Africa to live in cooler climates like Canada or Scandinavia.

Even in sunny countries, changing lifestyles mean more time is spent indoors in front of computers or in air-conditioned apartments, and vitamin D deficiency is becoming more frequent. Rickets—a childhood disease once relegated to medical history books—is reappearing in developed countries, and many children's hospitals now have rickets clinics. This appalling situation is easily preventable simply by ensuring that all infants and children receive a vitamin D supplement.

Vitamin D supplements: How much should I take?

Everyone can safely take the upper limit of vitamin D. This is 1,000 to 1,500 IU/day (25–37.5 mg) for infants; 2,500 to 3,000 IU/day (62.5–75 mg) for children aged one to eight; and 4,000 IU/day (100 mg) for those nine and older. Some people may need more than this to raise their blood level to the top end of the normal range, which some experts believe is optimal, since it is the level that can be achieved naturally by people who get reasonable amounts of sunshine all year round.[2]

To put vitamin D dosing into perspective, remember that anyone with pale (Caucasian) skin naturally makes at least 10,000 IU of vitamin D (250 mg) with twenty minutes of noonday summer sun exposure in a swimsuit—although someone with very dark skin might need up to two hours of sun exposure to make a similar amount. Common sense tells us that if 10,000 IU of vitamin D were seriously toxic, human beings would probably have died out as a species. Even the U.S. Institute of Medicine report on vitamin D commissioned by the Canadian and U.S. governments has grudgingly admitted that 10,000 IU is probably safe for most adults. However, some of us have evolved to cope better with the lower sun exposure in northern climates, and I find most people need quite a bit less than this to achieve good blood levels.

If you have been taking vitamin D regularly, you should eventually get your doctor to test your vitamin D level (25-hydroxyvitamin D). Do this in the middle of the winter, not the height of summer, when it may be temporarily elevated. The results of your blood test will show whether the amount you are taking is optimal for you. If it isn't, work with a knowledgeable health care provider to figure out how much more vitamin D you need to take to achieve a blood level in the upper end of the reference range, which is 75–250 nmol/L in Canada (30–100 ng/mL in the United States).

Should I stop taking vitamin D in the summer?

If twenty minutes of noonday sun is enough to generate 10,000 IU of vitamin D in Caucasian skin, what happens if you stay in the sun for longer? Will you continue making 10,000 IU every twenty minutes? It's unlikely. Ultraviolet radiation stimulates the manufacture of enzymes that control vitamin D metabolism, including an enzyme that breaks down excess vitamin D. Prolonged exposure to sunshine, therefore, will not cause toxic blood levels, although it does increase the risk of skin cancer. Supplements, on the other hand, do not appear to induce vitamin-D-controlling enzymes, so that blood levels can continue to rise, possibly to toxic levels, if excess vitamin D supplements are consumed. This is why testing your blood for vitamin D is so important.

I am often asked whether vitamin D supplements should be reduced or stopped in summer. I don't think so. By all means omit your vitamin D supplement if you have had twenty minutes in the sun that day without sunblock. But suppose you forget and take your supplement in addition to a little sunbathing? Don't worry. The vitamin-D-destroying enzymes you have made will make sure blood levels don't increase to toxic levels.

Vitamin E

The most important function for vitamin E is to protect fatty structures in the body from damage. The brain is approximately 60 per cent fat, and an increasing amount of research shows just how critical vitamin E is for brain health. Vitamin E and vitamin C also recycle one another, so you get better value from each one when you take both. Make sure the vitamin E you take is full spectrum—that is, contains all eight forms of vitamin E found naturally in food. Like the other fat-soluble vitamins, A, D, and K, vitamin E should be taken with a meal for proper absorption. Capsules vary in strength from approximately 400 to 550 IU daily. For most adults, one capsule daily is sufficient.

Avoid synthetic versions of vitamin E, such as dl-alpha tocopherol, although you can ignore the tiny amount that may be present in a multivitamin.

Vitamin K

Vitamin K has not been widely used as a supplement as it is thought to be relatively plentiful in food, and multivitamins have included vitamin K only relatively recently. As we saw in Chapter 7, vitamin K supplements may play a role in preventing arterial calcification, which is a risk factor for heart disease, stroke and dementia. You may need to supplement if you have a condition that affects absorption from the digestive tract, like Crohn's disease or celiac disease.

In the past there has been concern that too much vitamin K might over-activate blood clotting proteins and cause abnormal blood clotting. These fears are ungrounded—vitamin K controls whether blood clots but not how much it clots. Think of your car: gas is needed for it to start, but a full tank of gas does not mean the car will run faster.

Since no side effects are associated with vitamin K supplements, you may want to try them, especially if you have been diagnosed with osteoporosis or calcifications. Supplements usually contain 90–120 mg per capsule and should be taken at the same meal as vitamin D. Convenient supplements containing both 1,000 IU of vitamin D and 100–120 mg of vitamin K are now available.

Omega-3 fats (fish oil)

Today's fish oil supplements are much more pleasant to take than the cod liver oil we detested as children. Most fish oil is screened for mercury and other pollutants, and in the process, the fishy odour and taste is removed. Different brands of fish oil vary in their concentration of the two important long-chain fatty acids, EPA and DHA. Aim for a daily dose of approximately 500 mg of DHA and 750 mg of EPA. Although fish oil is available in capsules, the oil itself is easy to take and can be stirred into cold foods like yogurt or a smoothie.

Breastfed infants will get sufficient omega-3 fats if their mother is taking fish oil supplements. For children over one year, I recommend half the adult dose. Children nine and older can take the full adult dose.

Do we need calcium supplements?

The recommended daily intake of calcium is being gradually reduced across the developed world with the realization that modern diets are often overloaded with calcium. For years women have been told to take calcium supplements for bone health. However, research has found that supplements of calcium have little or no impact on bone health and could increase the risk of heart disease.[3]

North America has been slow to reduce the recommended daily requirement in line with current research, and recommendations still range from 1,000 to 1,200 mg daily from food and supplements combined. The European Union and the World Health Organization recommend 800 mg daily for men and women in any age group. This amount is not difficult to get from food, especially if you eat dairy products. Those who follow a vegan diet may be exceptions to this rule, and may therefore need a calcium supplement. However, many commercial non-dairy milk substitutes like almond or soy milk are often fortified with calcium and have a similar calcium content to cow's milk. Check your food intake using one of the many calcium calculators available on the Internet, for example, at www.osteoporosiscanada.ca.

If you need to supplement, I advise using a balanced calcium and magnesium supplement at a 2:1 ratio. Some forms of calcium and magnesium compete with each other for absorption. Using an amino acid– or protein-bound form, such as HVP (hydrolyzed vegetable protein) chelates, can overcome this.

Supplementing with magnesium

Apart from personal genetics, several factors increase the need for magnesium. The most important of these is stress, including the stress of pregnancy, other periods of rapid growth and heavy exercise. Excess dietary protein and fat, vitamin D, and high intakes of starchy carbohydrates (grains), sugar or alcohol increase magnesium needs. As we have seen, many commonly prescribed medications deplete magnesium. For all these reasons, magnesium can be one of the trickiest nutrients to optimally supplement.

Ultra-processed foods generally contain little or no magnesium, since most of it is lost during the refining process. The increased consumption of processed foods over the last several decades has therefore dramatically decreased dietary magnesium intake.[4] In addition, many high-fibre foods are also rich in compounds (e.g., phytates and oxalates) that bind magnesium and other minerals (calcium, zinc, manganese, etc.) and make them unavailable for absorption.[5] In this category are currently popular "superfoods" like chia and hemp seeds,[6] as well as wheat bran. I usually recommend avoiding these foods. While on paper they may be rich in minerals like calcium, magnesium and zinc, in my opinion their antinutrient content outweighs their benefits.

Don't be surprised if you start getting leg cramps after beginning to use these foods liberally in your diet—a sure sign they are depleting your magnesium.

Optimizing magnesium intake

Because bowel function relies on the contraction and relaxation of the muscles of the colon, too little magnesium will cause constipation (contraction without enough relaxation), while too much will over-relax the colon and cause loose stools. You can personalize your magnesium intake by gradually increasing the amount of supplemental magnesium until you have neither constipation nor diarrhea. This is called titrating magnesium to bowel tolerance.

The form of magnesium you take is important. I recommend using magnesium glycinate. Start with 100 mg at night before bed. After three days, begin to slowly increase your daily dose—by no more than half a pill (50 mg) every three days. Alternate additions between mornings and evening, until one to three soft, comfortable bowel movements are achieved each day. The reason for the slow increase of magnesium is to allow the gradual absorption and distribution of magnesium into all body tissues. If you take too much, too soon, you will certainly stimulate bowel muscle and eliminate constipation, but you will not achieve optimal tissue saturation, or provide the heart or brain with the constant supply of magnesium they need.

The amount of magnesium tolerated varies from one person to another. For some, 100 mg before bed may be all they can take, but others may need 300 or 400 mg twice a day to achieve bowel tolerance, especially if constipation has been a problem or they take medications that deplete magnesium. Rarely, some individuals may need even more. If stools become loose, cut back magnesium intake by 50 mg.

Using topical magnesium

While I do not think it is a substitute for regular oral magnesium, topical or transdermal forms of magnesium—absorbed through the skin—can also be useful. Commercial forms are available from health food stores as either gels or lotions.

A team of researchers at the Mayo Clinic asked forty women with fibromyalgia to spray magnesium chloride (31 per cent by weight in a proprietary blend of trace minerals) on their arms and legs, twice a day. After two and four weeks of treatment, patients reported a decrease in cramping, fatigue and joint and muscle pain. However, in this study the frequency of skin irritation led to a high dropout rate. Most of the commercial forms of topical magnesium are not pure magnesium but contain other minerals that can irritate and be very drying on the skin if used frequently. Some compounding pharmacies will make up magnesium gel or lotion to order. Ask for 15 per cent magnesium sulphate or magnesium chloride. I find that at this concentration, and without the addition of other trace minerals, there is little or no skin irritation.

Applied to arms or legs—peripheral circulation—magnesium gel is rapidly absorbed into the general circulation. Use about one teaspoon, spread on both hands, and rub evenly on forearms for shoulder tension or for sudden attacks of anxiety. Similarly, applied to calves and feet before bed, magnesium gel can help prevent restless legs or leg cramps.

Additional supplements to consider

The regime outlined above is a well-rounded general supplement regime for anyone wishing to preserve or enhance brain health. However, specific health problems or life stages may benefit from additional supplements. I usually suggest starting with the basic regime and waiting at least a month before adding in any of the supplements below.

Stress, including workplace stress, performance anxiety and PTSD

L-tyrosine. Take 1,500–2,000 mg on waking (empty stomach), and wait thirty minutes before eating. If stress is continuous throughout the day, an additional 1,000–1,500 mg can be taken midafternoon, two hours after food. Again, wait thirty minutes before eating. For working mothers, who generally arrive home to the busiest part of their day, I usually recommend taking this second dose of tyrosine just before leaving work. *Note:* Tyrosine supplements are recommended for adults only as there is no data on their use in children.

L-theanine. 250 mg in the morning and again before bed can be calming and help reduce excessive worry and anxiety. It is very helpful for "busy brain syndrome" or brain overload due to heavy employment demands. Take 250 mg whenever you feel overwhelmed.

Note that often when you buy amino acids the label has the prefix "L" in front of the name. The "L" indicates that the amino acid in question is in the form used naturally by the body.

Insomnia

Important: Wear an eye mask, or create complete blackout in your bedroom.

L-theanine. If you worry about getting to sleep, you may be suffering from sleep anxiety. If so, 250 mg of L-theanine before bed helps switch off the brain and create the right conditions for sleep.

5-HTP. If additional magnesium and L-theanine do not solve sleep problems, try adding 5-HTP (5-hydroxytryptophan). 5-HTP is the precursor for serotonin, which in turn gets converted into melatonin. Start with 100 mg just before bed. If necessary, increase the dose by 50–100 mg every four or five days, up to 300 mg. If you persistently wake in the night, place 100 mg beside the bed with a glass of water, and take this when you wake.

Melatonin. Melatonin may be particularly helpful if you have a long history of insomnia. For maximum impact, take it sixty to ninety minutes before bedtime. As with some other nutrients, it is best to start with a low dose and find the minimum dose you need to induce sleep. Start with 1 mg, and increase intake every four to five days to find your ideal dose.

Melatonin and 5-HTP. When going through particularly stressful times, or if you have long-standing insomnia, you may benefit from taking melatonin as directed above, and then following it with 100 to 300 mg of 5-HTP just before bed. This can help you not only fall asleep, but stay asleep. But take only the minimum doses that you need to achieve a good night's sleep.

Pregnancy

Chapter 10 outlines the supplement and diet regime I recommend for any woman wishing to get pregnant. It should be continued throughout the pregnancy and while breastfeeding. Two nutrients need special consideration because their need increases as pregnancy progresses: vitamin C and magnesium. I recommend increasing vitamin C by 1 g per day in the second trimester and again in the third trimester, to a total of 2 g twice a day.

Increase intake of magnesium by 50 mg any day bowels have been sluggish. Constipation and leg cramps are *not* a normal part of pregnancy but probably indicate the need for extra magnesium.

Attention deficit hyperactivity disorder (ADHD)

L-theanine (adults and children). Take 250 mg in the morning and again before bed. Children can benefit from an extra 250 mg before settling down to homework, while adults will find it helpful any time they feel overwhelmed.

L-tyrosine (adults only). Take as outlined above for stress.

Concussion or stroke recovery

All the supplements recommended for stress can be helpful.

Citicoline. 500–1,000 mg twice a day for memory recovery.

Memory improvement

L-tyrosine. Take as outlined for stress. Important for word recall and verbal fluency.

Citicoline. 500–1,000 mg twice a day.

Taking nutritional supplements: Information, misinformation and confusion

While the grocery store is familiar territory, a trip to buy vitamins may be an entirely new experience. Health food stores can be challenging places to navigate, and your first visit may be overwhelming. Faced with shelves and shelves of nutritional supplements—different brands, different dosages, different combinations of vitamins and minerals—how do you choose?

Rule number one is to be careful where you get advice. For example, don't rely only on store assistants to point you in the right direction. Remember, it's their job to sell you something—anything—and their advice is not impartial. It is also wise to avoid buying from a friend or neighbour selling supplements. These home-based businesses usually involve multilevel marketing schemes, in which the person selling you vitamins is making a profit not only from sales, but also from recruiting new salespeople to join the parent company. For every new distributor they recruit, they get a percentage of that person's sales. The products may be of good quality, but they are invariably overpriced, and you can probably buy similar products at a lower cost at your local health food store.

Not all these home businesses are legitimate, either. If the money is made primarily from sales of products, the business may be lawful. But if profits are made from recruiting other salespeople and supplying them with products, it's a pyramid scheme. Pyramid schemes are illegal in both Canada and the United States. Also remember that all the flyers and pamphlets you are given or pick up in stores are promotional materials: take any claims they make for a product with a grain of salt.

The trouble with Dr. Google

We all do it—turn to Dr. Google for health care advice. But beware of relying on the Internet for genuine information on nutritional supplements. While there are certainly excellent sites if you know where to look, much material is contradictory and confusing.

For example, a quick check shows that some medical websites suggest that the safe upper limit for daily intake of vitamin D is 2,000 IU.[7] This is incorrect. Both Health Canada and the Institute of Medicine in the United States have set 4,000 IU as the tolerable upper intake level (UL) for adults and all children from the age of nine.[8] As we have seen, the UL of a nutrient is defined as the amount you can take long term *without* supervision or blood tests, and with a negligible chance of side effects. However, at the time of writing the Mayo Clinic's website suggests that if you take more than 600 IU a day you should be supervised by a doctor.[9]

It's not just the public that can be misled by such confusing advice. One study in 2010 found that medical students relied heavily on searching for medical information on Google and Wikipedia.[10] Wikipedia is a free encyclopedia where anyone can write about anything. While some of its information is reliable, even Wikipedia admits that some articles can be complete rubbish. The problem is that you do not know the background or expertise of those making entries, since they are allowed to remain anonymous. Wikipedia claims that by allowing readers to revise what's posted, any errors will be edited out by more knowledgeable contributors and that this process will keep entries factually correct. Nice in theory, but it doesn't always work that way.

Bully tactics and the spread of false information

Because there is no peer review on Wikipedia, the editing process can result in "revision wars" between writers with different points of view. Some entries may be edited thousands of times an hour—you can find out how often by clicking on the tab marked "View history" at the top of an entry. You will get a list of the timing of all revisions and see what has been edited out. While some of these edits are genuine efforts to improve a topic and provide more up-to-date or accurate information, the system does provide a golden opportunity for anyone with an axe to grind who wants to push a specific agenda by spreading misinformation or "alternative facts."

When French composer Maurice Jarre died in 2009, Shane Fitzgerald, an Irish university student, saw a golden opportunity to test how easy it might be to disseminate false information through Wikipedia. As soon as he heard the announcement of Jarre's death he posted a quotation purportedly from Jarre himself: "Music was my life, music brought me to life, and music is how I will be remembered long after I leave this life. When I die there will be a final waltz playing in my head, that only I can hear." But Jarre never said any such thing. Fitzgerald had invented the quote.

Moderators at Wikipedia quickly removed the quote because its source was unclear. But Fitzgerald reposted it. Again, Wikipedia editors took it down, but Fitzgerald was persistent: every time Wikipedia moderators removed the quotation, he doggedly reinstated it. Using these bully tactics, he managed to keep the quotation on the website long enough for major news outlets to seize on it. Multiple reputable newspapers quoted it in their obituaries of Jarre.[11] Fitzgerald had not expected this outcome. He had thought his made-up unattributed quote might end up on some blogs and other amateur websites but not in quality mainstream newspapers. Don't they check facts?

After a few weeks, he contacted the newspapers and told them what he had done. Only one, the *Guardian* in the U.K., published a correction. This is just one small example of how a fact that is not a fact can become firmly established and take on an Internet life of its own.

The difference between opinion and evidence

The truth is that we have to be on guard when searching the Internet for reliable information on any topic. This applies equally to information about vitamins and other nutritional supplements. Very few reporters have the time, in-depth knowledge or interest to dig deep when reporting either positive or negative research findings. Making sense of different media reports on nutrition can leave you feeling concerned and exasperated, since they so often contradict each other.

At the Harvard T.H. Chan School of Public Health, they understand your frustration. The school's website points out that not all studies that get published are well designed. Badly designed studies deserve no attention, they say, as the results are likely to be inconclusive or even incorrect.[12] But not everyone reading the study has the in-depth knowledge needed to objectively critique the study, and its strengths and weaknesses. It is often sadly the case that badly designed studies are given a lot of media coverage, often by journalists who have simply read a press release and not the actual study. In fact, many publications that receive widespread media attention are not research at all but opinion pieces. And opinion pieces are just that—the opinion of the writers.

A typical example of the media confusing opinion with research appeared early in 2017. A thorough analysis of the many studies that have investigated the role of vitamin D in the prevention of upper respiratory tract infections clearly showed that low blood levels of vitamin D increased the risk of wintertime colds, flu and pneumonia. Although the protective effect of vitamin D was not huge, it was greatest in those with very low blood levels.[13] The authors concluded that public health measures should be taken to improve everyone's vitamin D status, especially in areas of the world most likely to be D-deficient in winter.

Newspaper headlines regarding that study were mostly positive, although many exaggerated the results. The BBC's webpage and newscast, for example, claimed that "vitamin D pills could stop colds or flu"—a huge overstatement. However, the same journal that published the study included an editorial by two other doctors who disputed the research, saying they were skeptical about its findings.[14] Some media reports chose to focus on the views expressed in the opinion piece rather than the research itself. "Study linking vitamin D to reduced cold and flu risk is too good to be true" was the headline in my daily newspaper. No wonder we get confused.

Naturally, insufficient vitamin D cannot be solely to blame for wintertime colds and flu, since the immune system is dependent on many other nutrients. But common sense tells us that if the incidence of these illnesses peaks in the winter months and falls off in the summer, lack of vitamin D could certainly play a role. In recent years, scientists have begun to clarify the many ways vitamin D contributes to the efficient functioning of our immune system. It seems logical to assume, therefore, that insufficient vitamin D would compromise our ability to fight infection.[15]

I am not arguing here against skepticism. In this age of hype and "alternative facts" it is important to remain vigilant against misinformation. But to be skeptical we need to be knowledgeable. We need to know how to critique research or find trustworthy experts who can do it for us. If we make snap judgments when we are not fully informed, we risk being labelled cynics, distrustful of *any* published research, from evidence for global warming to evidence for the benefits of vitamin D. What is important is that we keep an open mind.

But what about safety?

Reading some media reports, one might be forgiven for thinking that there was growing evidence nutritional supplements are dangerous and can cause serious health problems, even death. But the safety record of vitamins and mineral supplements is excellent, particularly when compared to the prescription drugs millions of people take every day. One Canadian study found that one in nine patients visiting hospital emergency departments was there because of an adverse reaction to a medication taken as prescribed. That's serious, particularly when we consider that 75 per cent of these adverse events were classified as moderate or severe.[16]

No such data exists for vitamins and minerals. We know from public records that very few deaths or serious adverse events have ever been attributed to vitamins taken as indicated either on the bottle or by a reputable health practitioner. Toddlers have unfortunately died after consuming toxic amounts of iron from adult multivitamins or iron supplements. But this is a preventable accident, not an adverse effect. Many multivitamins are sugar coated and seem like candy to a small child. I particularly advise against the use of "gummies," either for children or adults. Not only do they generally contain levels of some vitamins too low to be useful, they are meant to look and taste like candy and are particularly attractive to little kids.

When we talk about adverse events in the context of nutritional supplements, we should be careful to distinguish between symptoms that cause genuine health problems and those that are merely a nuisance. For example, excess magnesium intake from supplements can cause diarrhea. In people with modest magnesium requirements, quite a low dose could have this unwanted effect. But many people will benefit from and tolerate much higher doses, especially if they lead stressful lives or are taking certain medications.

If you follow the procedure outlined earlier in this chapter for optimizing your magnesium intake, increasing the amount you take slowly and by very small increments, you will end up with all the benefits of magnesium without this nuisance effect. The minor gastrointestinal distress that some people experience when taking supplements on an empty stomach can be overcome by consuming them with food. These nuisance effects should not be considered equivalent to an unwanted effect like liver toxicity, which is clearly serious.

Who decides what is safe?

Because there are ethical issues associated with conducting clinical trials for essential nutrients, safety levels for vitamins and minerals rely heavily on animal data and on long-term observation of populations using these products.[17] These studies are then reviewed periodically by committees to reach a consensus as to the tolerable upper intake level for a nutrient. Different regions have their own committees. In Europe, the European Food Safety Authority is the responsible body, while in North America it is the Institute of Medicine.

As we have seen, the UL is the dose of each essential nutrient we can take lifelong, with a high degree of confidence that we will not be harmed. For some nutrients like vitamin B12 and vitamin K there is no UL, since there is no evidence they are toxic at any level. As the U.S. Office of Dietary Supplements says, "no adverse effects associated with vitamin K consumption from food or supplements have been reported in humans or animals."[18] The same applies to B12: in healthy people, no toxic effects have been associated with high intakes.[19]

But we don't necessarily want excessive amounts—we want optimal intakes and a proper balance of nutrients. Optimal intakes allow the complex web of biochemical networks that controls our bodies and brains to function at its most efficient. If we are short of any single nutrient, our moods and our ability to think, sleep or remember will be compromised. We may take longer to heal after surgery. Our immune system will be inefficient and we may succumb more easily to colds and flu. Normal blood pressure or cholesterol levels may be difficult to maintain.

This is why it no longer surprises me when someone reports noticeable improvements in both their mental and physical well-being soon after they start a well-balanced supplement regime.

Essential means just that—essential!

Essential nutrients—the vitamins, minerals, essential fats and amino acids from protein—are indispensable to the functioning of the body: by definition it is impossible to be completely deficient in any of them and still be alive. However, it is not difficult to have an inadequate supply of one or more. Remember that recommended intakes exist because our health is compromised when we don't meet those daily targets.

After starting a supplement regime, try to take it consistently for at least a year. Then re-evaluate. You be the judge as to whether you have experienced any benefits. Has your energy increased, or your exercise tolerance improved? Are you sleeping better? Is your thinking clearer and word recall better? Have you survived the winter without a cold even though other family members have sniffled and coughed all winter long? Some of the beneficial effects of supplements are subtle at first, and not everyone will experience dramatic or immediate responses.

One of the aims of this book is to help you become a knowledge-able consumer. It is my hope that after reading this book you will find yourself more comfortable making choices about food, and especially about choosing supplements. If after a year you do not think your health has improved all that much, then the doses or balance of supplements you are taking may not be right for you, and it would be helpful to seek further advice from a knowledgeable practitioner.

At the very beginning this book I quoted E.O. Wilson, one of the world's preeminent biologists: "We are drowning in information" he says, "while starving for wisdom. The world henceforth will be run by synthe-sizers, people able to put together the right information at the right time, think critically about it, and make important choices wisely." I hope this book has helped the reader put together for themselves an approach to diet and supplements based on the best available evidence, and to make wise choices that will improve their mental and physical well-being.

APPENDIX

Fruit and Vegetable Diary

Week beginning _____

Mark each serving of fruit and vegetables you eat by ticking a single box. At the end of the week, total the number of boxes you have ticked, and write your score in the space provided.

FRUIT (for weight control, limit to three servings per day)					
1. 1/2 cup fruit juice	☐	☐	☐	☐	☐
2. 1/2 cup tinned fruit	☐	☐	☐	☐	☐
3. 1 medium banana	☐	☐	☐	☐	☐
4. 1 medium slice of cantaloupe	☐	☐	☐	☐	☐
5. 1 cup watermelon	☐	☐	☐	☐	☐
6. 1 fresh apple or pear	☐	☐	☐	☐	☐
7. 1 apricot (large) or plum (large)	☐	☐	☐	☐	☐
8. 1/2 cup apple sauce	☐	☐	☐	☐	☐
9. 1/2 cup berries (no syrup) (fresh or frozen)	☐	☐	☐	☐	☐
10. 1/4 cup dried fruit (raisins, apricots, etc.)	☐	☐	☐	☐	☐
11. 1 orange, tangerine or 1/2 grapefruit	☐	☐	☐	☐	☐
12. 1/2 cup prunes or figs (cubed) (soaked, no sugar)	☐	☐	☐	☐	☐
13. 1 peach or nectarine	☐	☐	☐	☐	☐
14. 1 cup pineapple (cubed)	☐	☐	☐	☐	☐

VEGETABLES (minimum three servings per day; no maximum)					
1. 1/2 glass vegetable juice (tomato, V8, etc.)	☐	☐	☐	☐	☐
2. 1/2 cup fresh, frozen or tinned peas or beans (lima, green, etc.)	☐	☐	☐	☐	☐
3. 1/2 cup broccoli or cauliflower	☐	☐	☐	☐	☐
4. 1 medium onion or 3 spring onions	☐	☐	☐	☐	☐
5. 1 medium tomato, or red or green pepper	☐	☐	☐	☐	☐
6. 1/2 cup cooked carrots	☐	☐	☐	☐	☐
7. 1 medium potato or medium yam	☐	☐	☐	☐	☐
8. 1 cup lettuce or mixed salad vegetables	☐	☐	☐	☐	☐
9. 1/2 cup cooked spinach or other greens	☐	☐	☐	☐	☐
10. 1 cup spinach (uncooked)	☐	☐	☐	☐	☐
11. 1/2 cup tomato sauce (i.e., spaghetti or pizza)	☐	☐	☐	☐	☐
12. 1 ear of corn (fresh) or 1/2 cup frozen or canned	☐	☐	☐	☐	☐
13. 1/2 cup tofu or soybeans	☐	☐	☐	☐	☐
14. 1/2 cup eggplant, zucchini, squash or pumpkin	☐	☐	☐	☐	☐
15. 1/2 cup cabbage or coleslaw	☐	☐	☐	☐	☐
16. 1 medium raw carrot or 4 large carrot sticks	☐	☐	☐	☐	☐
17. 1 stick of celery	☐	☐	☐	☐	☐
18. 1/2 cup bean or alfalfa sprouts	☐	☐	☐	☐	☐
19. 1/2 cup beets	☐	☐	☐	☐	☐
20. 1/2 cup beans or lentils (dried)	☐	☐	☐	☐	☐
21. 1 cup vegetable, lentil or bean soup	☐	☐	☐	☐	☐

Total score (for the week)	

HOW DID YOU RATE?

56–70	***Excellent.*** You are certainly taking healthy eating guidelines to heart and are eating the eight to ten servings of fruit and vegetables a day recommended for optimal health. If you maintain this level of consumption consistently, you should see your efforts repaid in the long term with a stronger immune system, slower aging and a reduced risk of major health problems such as cancer and heart disease. Congratulations.

35–55   ***Good.*** Your fruit and vegetable intake is above average and meets the *minimum* now considered necessary for good health. Try to maintain or improve on this. Choose dark green and orange vegetables, and orange fruits like cantaloupe and citrus, more often for maximum benefit.

21–34   ***Fair.*** Although you may think you are eating enough fruit and vegetables, your intake is lower than the recommended minimum five servings a day. Plan to have fruit or carrot sticks as a mid-morning or afternoon snack, and on days when it is difficult to get enough fresh produce, drink vegetable juice to supplement your intake.

20 or less ***Poor.*** Vegetables and fruit are key to staying healthy and avoiding the diseases associated with aging, such as heart disease, eye disease, cancer, diabetes and dementia.

Note: For maximum absorption of the phytochemicals that give fruits and vegetables much of their health benefits, always remember to eat them with a little fat.

Acknowledgements

I am enormously grateful to friends and colleagues for many helpful discussions in the development of this book. I would especially like to thank Drs. Nadine Bukmuz, Linda Rapson and Anne Marie Mingiardi, who were kind enough to read various drafts of the manuscript. Their thoughtful comments and suggestions have been invaluable.

A special thanks to my always encouraging agent, Beverley Slopen, and to my editor at HarperCollins, Patrick Crean, who helped to steer the book from proposal to completion. His good-humoured enthusiasm and steady guidance kept me on track as the work unfolded. I am grateful, too, to Alan Shar for his invaluable help with research.

I also want to acknowledge those who allowed me to tell their stories. Although individuals' names have been changed to protect their privacy, these stories are real, and I hope they enrich the book. Finally, during the writing of this book I have had tremendous encouragement and support from my family. Thank you, Oliver and Linda, for the delicious salmon dinners that were often Sunday evening lifesavers.

Endnotes

Introduction

1 World Health Organization, "Dementia," fact sheet, April 2016, www.who.int /mediacentre/factsheets/fs362/en.

2 Alzheimer Society of Canada, "Dementia Numbers in Canada," www.alzheimer .ca/en/About-dementia/What-is-dementia/Dementia-numbers.

3 S. Gillette Guyonnet et al., "IANA Task Force on Nutrition and Cognitive Decline with Aging," *Journal of Nutrition, Health and Aging* 11, 2 (2007): 132–52.

4 K.M. Adams et al., "Nutrition Education in U.S. Medical Schools: Latest Update of a National Survey," *Academic Medicine* 85, 9 (2010): 1537–42.

5 Health Canada, Canadian Community Health Survey, Cycle 2.2, Nutrition (2004), http://www.hc-sc.gc.ca/fn-an/surveill/nutrition/commun/index-eng .php; Scientific Report of the 2015 Dietary Advisory Committee, http://www .health.gov/dietaryguidelines/2015-scientific-report; R.S. Sebastian et al., "Older Adults Who Use Vitamin/Mineral Supplements Differ from Nonusers in Nutrient Intake Adequacy and Dietary Attitudes," *Journal of the American Dietetic Association* 107, 8 (2007): 1322–32.

6 Standing Senate Committee on Social Affairs, Science and Technology, *Obesity in Canada—A Whole-of-Society Approach for a Healthier Canada*, March 2016, http://www.parl.gc.ca/content/sen/committee/421/SOCI /Reports/2016-02-25_Revised_report_Obesity_in_Canada_e.pdf.

7 B.T. Burton, ed., *Heinz Handbook of Nutrition* (New York: McGraw-Hill, 1959).

8 M. Fenech et al., "Nutrigenetics and Nutrigenomics: Viewpoints on the Current Status and Applications in Nutrition Research and Practice," *Journal of Nutrigenetics and Nutrigenomics* 4, 2 (2011): 69–89.

9 E.M. Bik, "The Hoops, Hopes, and Hypes of Microbiome Research," *Yale Journal of Biology and Medicine* 89, 3 (2016): 363–73.

Chapter 1: A Journey across Time

1 A. Mobley et al., "A Survey on Data Reproducibility in Cancer Research Provides Insights into Our Limited Ability to Translate Findings from the Laboratory to the Clinic," *PLOS ONE* 8, 5 (2013): e63221.

2 J.D. Van Horn et al., "Mapping Connectivity Damage in the Case of Phineas Gage," *PLOS ONE* 7, 5 (2012): e37454.

3 R. Hooke, "Micrographia: Some Physiological Descriptions of Minute Bodies Made by Magnifying Glasses with Observations and Inquiries Thereupon," 1667, http:// www.gutenberg.org.

Chapter 2: Nature versus Nurture

1 S. Jinno, "Aging Affects New Cell Production in the Adult Hippocampus: A Quantitative Anatomic Review," *Journal of Chemical Neuroanatomy* 76, Part B (2016): 64–67.

2 B. Kolb and I.Q. Whishaw, *Fundamentals of Human Neuropsychology*, 5th ed. (New York: Worth Publishers, 2003).

3 S. Chen et al., "Reinstatement of Long-Term Memory Following Erasure of Its Behavioral and Synaptic Expression in *Aplysia*," *eLife*, November 17, 2014, e03896.

4 P.M. Dash et al., "Molecular Activity Underlying Working Memory," *Learning and Memory* 14 (2007): 554–63.

5 D. Gilbert, interviewed by H. Reese, "Psychology: 'An Owner's Manual for Your Own Mind,'" *Atlantic*, March 11, 2014, https://www.theatlantic.com/education /archive/2014/03/psychology-an-owner-s-manual-for-your-own-mind/284329.

6 K.C. Berridge and M.L. Kringelbach, "Building a Neuroscience of Pleasure and Well-being," *Psychology of Well-Being* 1, 1 (2011): 1–3.

7 A.J. Oswald and E. Proto, "National Happiness and Genetic Distance: A Cautious Exploration," IZA discussion paper no. 8300, July 2014, http://ftp.iza.org/dp8300 .pdf.

8 L.D. Kubzansky and R.C. Thurston, "Emotional Vitality and Incident Coronary Heart Disease: Benefits of Healthy Psychological Functioning," *Archives of General Psychiatry* 64, 12 (2007): 1393–401.

9 M.J. Lambiase et al., "Positive Psychological Health and Stroke Risk: The Benefits of Emotional Vitality," *Health Psychology* 34, 10 (2015): 1043–6; H. Achat et al., "Optimism and Depression As Predictors of Physical and Mental Health Functioning: The Normative Aging Study," *Annals of Behavioral Medicine* 22, 2 (2000): 127–30.

10 L.D. Kubzansky et al., "Early Manifestations of Personality and Adult Health: A Life Course Perspective," *Health Psychology* 28, 3 (2009): 364–72.

11 M. Mazza et al., "Affective and Cognitive Empathy in Adolescents with Autism Spectrum Disorder," *Frontiers in Human Neuroscience* 8 (2014): 791.

12 O. Schunke et al., "Mirror Me: Imitative Responses in Adults with Autism," *Autism* 20, 2 (2016): 134–44.

13 B. Chakrabarti et al., "Genes Related to Sex Steroids, Neural Growth, and Social-Emotional Behavior Are Associated with Autistic Traits, Empathy, and Asperger Syndrome," *Autism Research* 2, 3 (2009): 157–77.

14 P.L. Lockwood et al., "Neurocomputational Mechanisms of Prosocial Learning and Links to Empathy," *Proceedings of the National Academy of Sciences of the USA* 113, 35 (2016): 9763–68.

15 Canadian Council on Learning, *Bullying in Canada—How Intimidation Affects Learning*, March 20, 2008, http://en.copian.ca/library/research/ccl/bullying _in_canada/bullying_in_canada.pdf.

16 P. Stavrinides et al., "Bullying and Empathy: A Short-Term Longitudinal Investigation," *Educational Psychology* 30, 7 (2010): 793–802.

17 A. Duncan and C. Miller, "The Impact of an Abusive Family Context on Childhood Animal Cruelty and Adult Violence," *Aggression and Violent Behavior* 7, 4 (2002): 365–83.

18 A. Kimberly et al., "Promoting Children's Prosocial Behaviors in School: Competence of School-Aged Children. Impact of the 'Roots of Empathy' Program on the Social and Emotional Competence of School-Aged Children," *School Mental Health* 4 (2012): 1–21.

19 O. Van der Rest et al., "Dietary Patterns, Cognitive Decline, and Dementia: A Systematic Review," *Advances in Nutrition* 6, 2 (2015): 154–68.

Chapter 3: The Nutrition-Cognition Connection

1 T.C. Durazzo et al., "Smoking and Increased Alzheimer's Disease Risk: A Review of Potential Mechanisms," *Alzheimer's and Dementia* 10, S3 (2014): S122–45.

2 S. Haller et al., "Acute Caffeine Administration Impact on Working Memory -Related Brain Activation and Functional Connectivity in the Elderly: A BOLD and Perfusion MRI Study," *Neuroscience* 250 (2013): 364–71.

3 Harvard Medical School, "Glycemic Index and Glycemic Load for 100+ Foods," last updated August 27, 2015, http://www.health.harvard.edu/diseases-and-conditions/glycemic_index_and_glycemic_load_for_100_foods (accessed April 1, 2017).

4 E.R. Seaquist, "The Impact of Diabetes on Cerebral Structure and Function," *Psychosomatic Medicine* 77, 6 (2015): 616–21.

5 R. Elango et al., "Evidence That Protein Requirements Have Been Significantly Underestimated," *Current Opinion in Clinical Nutrition and Metabolic Care* 13, 1 (2010): 52–57.

6 T.B. Symons et al., "A Moderate Serving of High-Quality Protein Maximally Stimulates Skeletal Muscle Protein Synthesis in Young and Elderly Subjects," *Journal of the American Dietetic Association* 109, 9 (2009): 1582–86.

7 R.J. Wurtman, "Behavioural Effects of Nutrients," *Lancet* 1, 8334 (1983): 1145–47.

8 H.R. Lieberman et al., "Mood, Performance and Pain Sensitivity: Changes Induced by Food Constituents," *Journal of Psychiatric Research* 17, 2 (1982–83): 135–45.

9 R.P. Patrick and B.N. Ames, "Vitamin D and the Omega-3 Fatty Acids Control Serotonin Synthesis and Action, Part 2: Relevance for ADHD, Bipolar Disorder, Schizophrenia, and Impulsive Behavior," *FASEB Journal* 29, 6 (2015): 2207–22.

10 M. de Lorgeril and P. Salen, "New Insights into the Health Effects of Dietary Saturated and Omega-6 and Omega-3 Polyunsaturated Fatty Acids," *BMC Medicine* 10 (2012): 50.

11 Patrick and Ames, "Vitamin D and the Omega-3 Fatty Acids."

12 D. Kromhout, "Where the Latest U.S. Dietary Guidelines Are Heading," *BMJ* 35 (2015): h4034.

13 P.W. Siri-Tarino et al., "Meta-analysis of Prospective Cohort Studies Evaluating the Association of Saturated Fat with Cardiovascular Disease," *American Journal of Clinical Nutrition* 91, 3 (2010): 535–46.

14 J. Yerushalmy and H.E. Hilleboe, "Fat in the Diet and Mortality from Heart Disease: A Methodologic Note," *New York State Journal of Medicine* 57 (1957): 2343–54.

15 C. Hryhorczuk et al., "Dampened Mesolimbic Dopamine Function and Signaling by Saturated but Not Monounsaturated Dietary Lipids," *Neuropsychopharmacology* 41, 3 (2016): 811–21.

16 L. Morgan et al., "Comparison of the Effects of Four Commercially Available Weight-Loss Programmes on Lipid-Based Cardiovascular Risk Factors," *Public Health Nutrition* 23 (2008): 1–9.

17 J.W. Rankin and A.D. Turpyn, "Low Carbohydrate, High Fat Diet Increases C-Reactive Protein during Weight Loss," *Journal of the American College of Nutrition* 26, 2 (2007): 163–69.

18 R. Schmidt et al., "Early Inflammation and Dementia: A 25-Year Follow-up of the Honolulu-Asia Aging Study," *Annals of Neurology* 52, 2 (2002): 168–74.

19 B.A. Golomb and A.K. Bui, "A Fat to Forget: Trans Fat Consumption and Memory," *PLOS ONE* 10, 6 (2015): e0128129.

20 Grocery Manufacturers Association, Executive summary of GMA's Food Additive Petition, August 5, 2015, Center for Science in the Public Interest, http://cspinet.org/new/pdf/gma_trans_fat_fap_executive_summary_8-5-15.pdf.

Chapter 4: Vitamins, Minerals and Brain Function

1 E.V. McCollum, *A History of Nutrition* (Cambridge, MA: Riverside Press, 1957); S.A. Goldblith and M.A. Joslyn, eds., *Milestones in Nutrition*, vol. 2 (Westport, CT: AVI Publishing, 1964).

2 L.A. Bazzano et al., "Effects of Low-Carbohydrate and Low-Fat Diets: A Randomized Trial," *Annals of Internal Medicine* 161, 5 (2014): 309–18.

3 J.P. Blass, "Brain Metabolism and Brain Disease: Is Metabolic Deficiency the Proximate Cause of Alzheimer Dementia?" *Journal of Neuroscience Research* 66 (2001): 851–56.

4 D. Mulleman and P. Goupille, "Medical Mystery: Extensive Ecchymosis—The Answer," *New England Journal of Medicine* 354, 4 (2006): 419–20.

5 Y. Wang et al., "Effects of Vitamin C and Vitamin D Administration on Mood and Distress in Acutely Hospitalized Patients," *American Journal of Clinical Nutrition* 98, 3 (2013): 705–11.

6 B.J. Kaplan et al., "A Randomised Trial of Nutrient Supplements to Minimise Psychological Stress after a Natural Disaster," *Psychiatry Research* 228, 3 (2015): 373–79.

7 D.O. Kennedy et al., "Effects of High-Dose B Vitamin Complex with Vitamin C and Minerals on Subjective Mood and Performance in Healthy Males," *Psychopharmacology* (Berlin) 211, 1 (2010): 55–68.

8 J.P. Spencer, "Food for Thought: The Role of Dietary Flavonoids in Enhancing Human Memory, Learning and Neurocognitive Performance," *Proceedings of the Nutrition Society* 67, 2 (2008): 238–52.

9 P.H. Warnke et al., "The Ongoing Battle against Multi-resistant Strains: In-vitro

Inhibition of Hospital-Acquired MRSA, VRE, *Pseudomonas*, ESBL *E. coli* and *Klebsiella* Species in the Presence of Plant-Derived Antiseptic Oils," *Journal of Cranio-maxillo-facial Surgery* 41, 4 (2013): 321–26.

10 O. Oyebode et al., "Fruit and Vegetable Consumption and All-Cause, Cancer and CVD Mortality: Analysis of Health Survey for England Data," *Journal of Epidemiology and Community Health* 68, 9 (2014): 856–62.

11 S. Seetharaman et al., "Blood Glucose, Diet-Based Glycemic Load and Cognitive Aging among Dementia-Free Older Adults," *Journals of Gerontology, Series A, Biological Sciences and Medical Sciences* 70, 4 (2015): 471–79.

12 M.C. Morris et al., "MIND Diet Slows Cognitive Decline with Aging," *World Review of Nutrition and Dietetics* 115 (2016): 98–108.

13 G.H. Beaton and E.W. McHenry, eds. "Nutrition and Public Health," *Quarterly Bulletin of the Health Organization of the League of Nations* 1 (1935): 1–152.

14 Health Canada, "Dietary Reference Intakes," January 23, 2006, http://www.hc-sc .gc.ca/fn-an/nutrition/reference/table/ref_macronutr_tbl-eng.php (accessed August 31, 2015).

15 J. Bauer et al., "Evidence-Based Recommendations for Optimal Dietary Protein Intake in Older People: A Position Paper from the PROT-AGE Study Group," *Journal of the American Medical Directors Association* 14, 8 (2013): 542–59.

Chapter 5: Alzheimer's and Dementia: Our Greatest Fears

1 E. Dawkins and D.H. Small, "Insights into the Physiological Function of the β-Amyloid Precursor Protein: Beyond Alzheimer's Disease," *Journal of Neurochemistry* 129, 5 (2014): 756–69.

2 T.A. Pascoal et al., "Amyloid-β and Hyperphosphorylated Tau Synergy Drives Metabolic Decline in Preclinical Alzheimer's Disease," *Molecular Psychiatry* 22, 2 (2017): 306–11.

3 L.S. Schneider, "Estrogen and Dementia: Insights from the Women's Health Initiative Memory Study," *JAMA* 291, 24 (2004): 3005–7.

4 J.P. Reis et al., "Subclinical Atherosclerotic Calcification and Cognitive Functioning in Middle-Aged Adults: The CARDIA Study," *Atherosclerosis* 231, 1 (2013): 72–77.

5 S. Gauthier et al., "Mild Cognitive Impairment," *Lancet* 367 (2006): 1262–70.

6 G.P. Morris et al., "Inconsistencies and Controversies Surrounding the Amyloid Hypothesis of Alzheimer's Disease," *Acta Neuropathologica Communications* 2 (2014): 135.

7 C.B. Parker, "Scientific Evidence Does Not Support the Brain Game Claims, Stanford Scholars Say," Stanford News Service, October 20, 2014, http://news .stanford.edu/pr/2014/pr-brain-games-carstensen-102014.html.

8 L. Oberman and A. Pascual-Leone, "Changes in Plasticity across the Lifespan: Cause of Disease and Target for Intervention," *Progress in Brain Research* 207 (2013): 91–120.

9 EClipSE Collaborative Members, "Education, the Brain and Dementia: Neuroprotection or Compensation?" *Brain* 133, 8 (2010): 2210–16.

10 E. Rieman et al., "Brain Imaging and Fluid Biomarker Analysis in Young Adults at Genetic Risk for Autosomal Dominant Alzheimer's Disease in the Presenilin 1 E280A Kindred: A Case-Control Study," *Lancet Neurology* 11, 12 (2012): 1048–56.

11 World Health Organization, *Tobacco and Dementia*, June 2014, http://apps.who .int/iris/bitstream/10665/128041/1/WHO_NMH_PND_CIC_TKS_14.1_eng.pdf.

12 B. Shakersain et al., "Prudent Diet May Attenuate the Adverse Effects of Western Diet on Cognitive Decline," *Alzheimer's and Dementia* 12, 2 (2016): 100–109.

13 S.M. de la Monte and J.R. Wand, "Alzheimer's Disease Is Type 3 Diabetes— Evidence Reviewed," *Journal of Diabetes Science and Technology* 2, 6 (2008): 1101–13.

14 S. Berntsen et al., "Alcohol Consumption and Mortality in Patients with Mild Alzheimer's Disease: A Prospective Cohort Study," *BMJ Open* 5, 12 (2015): e007851.

15 J.J. Iliff et al., "A Paravascular Pathway Facilitates CSF Flow through the Brain Parenchyma and the Clearance of Interstitial Solutes, Including Amyloid β," *Science Translational Medicine* 4, 147 (2012): 147ra111.

16 J. Zhang and Q. Liu, "Cholesterol Metabolism and Homeostasis in the Brain," *Protein and Cell* 6, 4 (2015): 254–64.

17 U.S. Food and Drug Administration, "Controlling Cholesterol with Statins," February 29, 2012, http://www.fda.gov/ForConsumers/ConsumerUpdates /ucm293330.htm (accessed December 10, 2016).

18 B.L. Strom et al., "Statin Therapy and Risk of Acute Memory Impairment," *JAMA Internal Medicine* 175, 8 (2015): 1399–405.

19 L. Spinney, "Alzheimer's Disease: The Forgetting Gene," *Nature* 510 (2014): 26–28.

20 E. Hjorth et al., "Omega-3 Fatty Acids Enhance Phagocytosis of Alzheimer's Disease-Related Amyloid-β42 by Human Microglia and Decrease Inflammatory Markers," *Journal of Alzheimer's Disease* 35, 4 (2013): 697–713.

21 J. Nishihira et al., "Associations between Serum Omega-3 Fatty Acid Levels and Cognitive Functions among Community-Dwelling Octogenarians in Okinawa, Japan: The KOCOA Study," *Journal of Alzheimer's Disease* 51, 3 (2016): 857–66.

22 A. Oulhaj et al., "Omega-3 Fatty Acid Status Enhances the Prevention of Cognitive Decline by B Vitamins in Mild Cognitive Impairment," *Journal of Alzheimer's Disease* 50, 2 (2016): 547–57.

23 N. Tajuddin et al., "Neuroinflammation and Neurodegeneration in Adult Rat Brain from Binge Ethanol Exposure: Abrogation by Docosahexaenoic Acid," *PLOS ONE* 9, 7 (2014): e101223.

24 M.S. Morris et al., "Folate and Vitamin B-12 Status in Relation to Anemia, Macrocytosis, and Cognitive Impairment in Older Americans in the Age of Folic Acid Fortification," *American Journal of Clinical Nutrition* 85 (2007): 193–200.

25 A. Vogiatzoglou et al., "Vitamin B12 Status and Rate of Brain Volume Loss in Community-Dwelling Elderly," *Neurology* 71, 11 (2008): 826–32.

26 D. Bunce et al., "Apolipoprotein E, B Vitamins, and Cognitive Function in Older Adults," *Journals of Gerontology, Series B, Psychological Sciences and Social Sciences* 60, 1 (2005): 41–48.

27 A.D. Smith et al., "Homocysteine-Lowering by B Vitamins Slows the Rate of

Accelerated Brain Atrophy in Mild Cognitive Impairment: A Randomized Controlled Trial," *PLOS ONE* 5, 9 (2010): e12244.

28 D.J. Llewellyn et al., "Vitamin D and Risk of Cognitive Decline in Elderly Persons," *Archives of Internal Medicine* 170 (2010): 1135–41.

29 T.J. Littlejohns et al., "Vitamin D and the Risk of Dementia and Alzheimer Disease," *Neurology* 83, 10 (2014): 920–28.

30 I. Karakis et al., "Association of Serum Vitamin D with the Risk of Incident Dementia and Subclinical Indices of Brain Aging: The Framingham Heart Study," *Journal of Alzheimer's Disease* 51, 2 (2016): 451–61.

31 M.T. Mizwicki et al., "1α,25-dihydroxyvitamin D3 and Resolvin D1 Retune the Balance between Amyloid-β Phagocytosis and Inflammation in Alzheimer's Disease Patients," *Journal of Alzheimer's Disease* 34, 1 (2013): 155–70.

32 J.D. Spence, "Metabolic Vitamin B12 Deficiency: A Missed Opportunity to Prevent Dementia and Stroke," *Nutrition Research* 36, 2 (2016): 109–16.

Chapter 6: This Is Your Brain on Stress

1   T.C. Russ, "Association between Psychological Distress and Mortality: Individual Participant Pooled Analysis of 10 Prospective Cohort Studies," *BMJ* 345 (2012): e4933.

2   F. Calabrese et al., "Neuronal Plasticity: A link between Stress and Mood Disorders," *Psychoneuroendocrinology* 34S (2009): S208–16.

3   A. Machado et al., "Chronic Stress As a Risk Factor for Alzheimer's Disease," *Reviews in the Neurosciences* 25, 6 (2014): 785–804.

4   A.F. Arnsten, "Stress Weakens Prefrontal Networks: Molecular Insults to Higher Cognition," *Nature Neuroscience* 18, 10 (2015): 1376–85.

5   C. Anacker et al., "Glucocorticoid-Related Molecular Signaling Pathways Regulating Hippocampal Neurogenesis," *Neuropsychopharmacology* 38, 5 (2013): 872–83.

6   L.S. Colzato et al., "Food for Creativity: Tyrosine Promotes Deep Thinking," *Psychological Research* 79, 5 (2015): 709–14.

7   A.W. Flaherty, "Frontotemporal and Dopaminergic Control of Idea Generation and Creative Drive," *Journal of Complementary Neurology* 493 (2005): 147–53.

8   L.S. Colzato et al., "Eating to Stop: Tyrosine Supplementation Enhances Inhibitory Control but Not Response Execution," *Neuropsychologia* 62 (2014): 398–402.

9   A. Hase et al., "Behavioral and Cognitive Effects of Tyrosine Intake in Healthy Human Adults," *Pharmacology, Biochemistry, and Behavior* 133 (2015): 1–6.

10 N.A. Coull et al., "Effect of Tyrosine Ingestion on Cognitive and Physical Performance Utilising an Intermittent Soccer Performance Test (iSPT) in a Warm Environment," *European Journal of Applied Physiology* 115, 2 (2015): 373–86.

11 C.A. Salter et al., "Dietary Tyrosine As an Aid to Stress Resistance among Troops," *Military Medicine* 154, 3 (1989): 144–46.

12 L. Cahill et al., "Vitamin C Deficiency in a Population of Young Canadian Adults," *American Journal of Epidemiology* 170, 4 (2009): 464–71.

13 M.L. Yew, "'Recommended Daily Allowances' for Vitamin C," *Proceedings of the National Academy of Sciences of the USA* 70, 4 (1973): 969–72.

14 A. Sadeghpour et al., "Impact of Vitamin C Supplementation on Post-Cardiac Surgery ICU and Hospital Length of Stay," *Anesthesiology and Pain Medicine* 5, 1 (2015): e25337.

15 A.E. Carrillo et al., "Vitamin C Supplementation and Salivary Immune Function Following Exercise-Heat Stress," *International Journal of Sports Physiology and Performance* 3, 4 (2008): 516–30.

16 A. Moshfegh et al., *What We Eat in America, NHANES 2005–2006*, 2009, U.S. Department of Agriculture, Agricultural Research Service, https://www.ars .usda.gov/SP2UserFiles/Place/80400530/pdf/0506/usual_nutrient_intake _vitD_ca_phos_mg_2005-06.pdf.

17 Health Canada, "Do Canadian Adults Meet Their Nutrient Requirements through Food Intake Alone?" 2012, http://www.hc-sc.gc.ca/fn-an/surveill /nutrition/commun/art-nutr-adult-eng.php#a33, (accessed November 25, 2015).

18 G. Grases et al., "Anxiety and Stress among Science Students: Study of Calcium and Magnesium Alterations," *Magnesium Research* 19, 2 (2006): 102–6.

19 K.A. Barbour et al., "Exercise As a Treatment for Depression and Other Psychiatric Disorders: A Review," *Journal of Cardiopulmonary Rehabilitation and Prevention* 27, 6 (2007): 359–67.

20 A.T. Ludlow et al., "Relationship between Physical Activity Level, Telomere Length, and Telomerase Activity," *Medicine and Science in Sports and Exercise* 40, 10 (2008): 1764–71.

21 A. Chiesa et al., "Mindfulness-Based Stress Reduction for Stress Management in Healthy People: A Review and Meta-analysis," *Journal of Alternative and Complementary Medicine* 15, 5 (2009): 593–600.

Chapter 7: Brain Injuries: Trauma and Stroke

1 H.S. Martland, "Punch Drunk," *JAMA* 91, 15 (1928): 1103–7.

2 A.C. McKee et al., "The Spectrum of Disease in Chronic Traumatic Encephalopathy," *Brain* 136, 1 (2013): 43–64.

3 J.M. Silver, T.W. McAllister and D.B. Arciniegas, "Depression and Cognitive Complaints Following Mild Traumatic Brain Injury," *American Journal of Psychiatry* 166 (2009): 653–61.

4 J.M. Stamm et al., "Age of First Exposure to Football and Later-Life Cognitive Impairment in Former NFL Players," *Neurology* 84, 11 (2015): 1114–20.

5 Z.Y. Kerr et al., "Concussion Symptoms and Return to Play Time in Youth, High School, and College American Football Athletes," *JAMA Pediatrics* 170, 7 (2016): 647–53.

6 D.J. Wiebe et al., "Identification and Validation of Prognostic Criteria for Persistence of Mild Traumatic Brain Injury-Related Impairment in the Pediatric Patient," *Pediatric Emergency Care* 28, 6 (2012): 498–502.

7 Quoted in M. Walker, "Debate on Youth Football and Concussions," *MedPage Today*, December 24, 2015, http://www.medpagetoday.com/Pediatrics /GeneralPediatrics/55426.

8   R.R. Leker and E. Shohami, "Cerebral Ischemia and Trauma-Different Etiologies Yet Similar Mechanisms: Neuroprotective Opportunities," *Brain Research, Brain Research Reviews* 39 (2002): 55–73.

9   "Same Symptoms, Different Cause: TIAs May Arise from Different Mechanisms," http://www.medscape.com/viewarticle/786270.

10 M. Houston et al., "The Role of Magnesium in Hypertension and Cardiovascular Disease," *Journal of Clinical Hypertension* (Greenwich, CT) 13, 11 (2011): 843–47.

11 W.W. Oppelt et al., "Magnesium Exchange between Blood and Cerebrospinal Fluid," *American Journal of Physiology* 205 (1963): 959–62.

12 Z. Ram et al., "Magnesium Sulfate Reverses Experimental Delayed Cerebral Vasospasm after Subarachnoid Hemorrhage in Rats," *Stroke* 22 (1991): 922–27.

13 K.W. Muir, "Magnesium for Neuroprotection in Ischaemic Stroke: Rationale for Use and Evidence of Effectiveness," *CNS Drugs* 15, 12 (2001): 921–30.

14 H. Morisaki et al., "Hypermagnesemia-Induced Cardiopulmonary Arrest before Induction of Anesthesia for Emergency Cesarean Section," *Journal of Clinical Anesthesia* 12, 3 (2000): 224–26.

15 V. Trapani et al., "Magnesium and the Yin-Yang Interplay in Apoptosis," in *Magnesium in the Central Nervous System*, ed. R. Vink and M. Nechifor (Adelaide, Australia: University of Adelaide Press, 2011), 85–98.

16 C-Y. Yang, "Calcium and Magnesium in Drinking Water and Risk of Death from Cerebrovascular Disease," *Stroke* 29 (1998): 411–14.

17 S.C. Larsson et al., "Dietary Magnesium Intake and Risk of Stroke: A Meta-analysis of Prospective Studies," *American Journal of Clinical Nutrition* 95, 2 (2012): 362–66.

18 T. Wahls et al., "Assessment of Dietary Adequacy for Important Brain Micronutrients in Patients Presenting to a Traumatic Brain Injury Clinic for Evaluation," *Nutritional Neuroscience* 17, 6 (2014): 252–59.

19 K.E. Saatman et al., "Acute Cytoskeletal Alterations and Cell Death Induced by Experimental Brain Injury Are Attenuated by Magnesium Treatment and Exacerbated by Magnesium Deficiency," *Journal of Neuropathology and Experimental Neurology* 60, 2 (2001): 183–94.

20 M.J. Berridge et al., "The Versatility and Universality of Calcium Signalling," *Nature Reviews in Molecular and Cellular Biology* 1 (2000): 11–21.

21 J.B Anderson and P.J. Klemmer, "Risk of High Dietary Calcium for Arterial Calcification in Older Adults," *Nutrients* 5, 10 (2013): 3964–74.

22 J. Adams and J. Pepping, "Vitamin K in the Treatment and Prevention of Osteoporosis and Arterial Calcification," *American Journal of Health-System Pharmacology* 62, 15 (2005): 1574–81.

23 Z.A. Fazeel and G. Fazeelath, "Efficacy of Vitamin K as a Supplement in Osteoporosis," *European Journal of Biotechnology and Bioscience* 2, 6 (2014): 25–29.

24 E. Theuwissen et al., "The Role of Vitamin K in Soft-Tissue Calcification," 3, 2 (2012): 166–73.

25 D. Bos et al., "Calcification in Major Vessel Beds Relates to Vascular Brain Disease," *Arteriosclerosis Thrombosis and Vascular Biology* 31, 10 (2011): 2331–37.

26 N. Inaba et al., "Low-Dose Daily Intake of Vitamin K(2) (Menaquinone-7) Improves Osteocalcin γ-Carboxylation: A Double-Blind, Randomized Controlled Trial," *Journal of Nutritional Science and Vitaminology* (Tokyo) 61, 6 (2015): 471–80.

27 M.K. Shea et al., "Association between Circulating Vitamin K1 and Coronary Calcium Progression in Community-Dwelling Adults: The Multi-Ethnic Study of Atherosclerosis," *American Journal of Clinical Nutrition* 98, 1 (2013): 197–208.

28 Linus Pauling Institute Micronutrient Information Center, Oregon State University, "Vitamin K," http://lpi.oregonstate.edu/mic/vitamins/vitamin-K.

29 M.H. Rabadi et al., "Intensive Nutritional Supplements Can Improve Outcomes in Stroke Rehabilitation," *Neurology* 71, 23 (2008): 1856–61.

30 D. Vauzour et al., "The Neuroprotective Potential of Flavonoids: A Multiplicity of Effects," *Genes and Nutrition* 3, 3–4 (2008): 115–26.

31 G.C. Chen et al., "Vitamin C Intake, Circulating Vitamin C and Risk of Stroke: A Meta-analysis of Prospective Studies," *Journal of the American Heart Association* 2, 6 (2013): e000329.

32 H. Dong et al., "Efficacy of Supplementation with B Vitamins for Stroke Prevention: A Network Meta-Analysis of Randomized Controlled Trials," *PLOS ONE* 10, 9 (2015): e0137533.

33 Wahls et al., "Assessment of Dietary Adequacy."

34 N.W. Liles et al., "Diversity and Severity of Adverse Reactions to Quinine: A Systematic Review," *American Journal of Hematology* 91, 5 (2016): 461–66.

35 F.W. Heaton et al., "External Factors Affecting Diurnal Variation in Electrolyte Excretion with Particular Reference to Calcium and Magnesium," *Clinica Chimica Acta* 8, 2 (1963): 246–54.

36 G. Scott et al., "Amyloid Pathology and Axonal Injury after Brain Trauma," *Neurology* 86, 9 (2016): 821–8.

37 K. Shinozuka et al., "Melatonin-Based Therapeutics for Neuroprotection in Stroke," *International Journal of Molecular Sciences* 14, 5 (2013): 8924–47.

38 S.H. Su et al., "Elevated C-Reactive Protein Levels May Be a Predictor of Persistent Unfavourable Symptoms in Patients with Mild Traumatic Brain Injury: A Preliminary Study," *Brain, Behavior and Immunity* 38 (2014): 111–17.

39 G. Block et al., "Vitamin C Treatment Reduces Elevated C-Reactive Protein," *Free Radical Biology and Medicine* 46, 1 (2009): 70–77.

40 D. Frankenfield, "Energy Expenditure and Protein Requirements after Traumatic Injury," *Nutrition in Clinical Practice* 21, 5 (2006): 430–37.

41 D.R. Hill and D.S. Newburg, "Clinical Applications of Bioactive Milk Components," *Nutrition Reviews* 2015 73(7): 463–76.

42 M.P. Lin et al., "'Life's Simple 7' and Long-Term Mortality after Stroke," *Journal of the American Heart Association* 4, 11 (2015): pii: e001470.

43 K. Matsushima et al., "Glucose Variability Negatively Impacts Long-Term Functional Outcome in Patients with Traumatic Brain Injury," *Journal of Critical Care* 27, 2 (2012): 125–31.

Chapter 8: Brain under Construction: Diet and Pregnancy

1   J.E. Harding et al., "The Nutritional Basis of the Fetal Origins of Adult Disease," *International Journal of Epidemiology* 30, 1 (2001): 15–23.
2   T. Pongcharoen et al., "Influence of Prenatal and Postnatal Growth on Intellectual Functioning in School-Aged Children," *Archives of Pediatrics and Adolescent Medicine* 166, 5 (2012): 411–16.
3   D. Almond and J. Currie, "Killing Me Softly: The Fetal Origins Hypothesis," *Journal of Economic Perspective* 25, 3 (2011): 153–72.
4   C.D. Byrne and D.I. Phillips, "Fetal Origins of Adult Disease: Epidemiology and Mechanisms," *Journal of Clinical Pathology* 53 (2000): 822–28.
5   R.S. Strauss, "Adult Functional Outcome of Those Born Small for Gestational Age: Twenty-Six-Year Follow-up of the 1970 British Birth Cohort," *JAMA* 283, 5 (2000): 625–32.
6   D.J.P. Barker, "The Malnourished Baby and Infant: Relationship with Type 2 Diabetes," *British Medical Bulletin* 60, 1(2001): 69–88.
7   P. Sable et al., "Maternal Micronutrients and Brain Global Methylation Patterns in the Offspring," *Nutrition and Neuroscience* 18 (2015): 30–36.
8   M. Lane et al., "Peri-Conception Parental Obesity, Reproductive Health, and Trans-generational Impacts," *Trends in Endocrinology and Metabolism* 26, 2 (2015): 84–90.
9   M.E. Pembrey et al., "Sex-Specific, Male-Line Transgenerational Responses in Humans," *European Journal of Human Genetics* 14 (2006): 159–66.
10 K.G. Harly et al., "Prenatal and Early Childhood Bisphenol A Concentrations and Behavior in School-Aged Children," *Environmental Research* 126 (2013): 43–50.
11 A. Baccarelli and V. Bollati, "Epigenetics and Environmental Chemicals," *Current Opinion in Pediatrics* 21, 2 (2009): 243–51.
12 J.L. Bolton and S.D. Bilbo, "Developmental Programming of Brain and Behavior by Perinatal Diet: Focus on Inflammatory Mechanisms," *Dialogues in Clinical Neuroscience* 16, 3 (2014): 307–20.
13 W.D. Lassek et al., "Linoleic and Docosahexaenoic Acids in Human Milk Have Opposite Relationships with Cognitive Test Performance in a Sample of 28 Countries," *Prostaglandins, Leukotrienes and Essential Fatty Acids* 91, 5 (2014): 195–201.
14 I.P. Tzanetakou et al., "Nutrition during Pregnancy and the Effect of Carbohydrates on the Offspring's Metabolic Profile: In Search of the 'Perfect Maternal Diet,'" *Open Cardiovascular Medicine Journal* 5 (2011): 103–9.
15 U. Nurmatov, G. Devereux and A. Sheikh, "Nutrients and Foods for the Primary Prevention of Asthma and Allergy: Systematic Review and Meta-analysis," *Journal of Allergy and Clinical Immunology* 127, 3 (2011): 724–33.
16 T.V. Stephens et al., "Protein Requirements of Healthy Pregnant Women during Early and Late Gestation Are Higher Than Current Recommendations," *Journal of Nutrition* 145, 1 (2015): 73–78.
17 M. M. Mamerow et al., "Dietary Protein Distribution Positively Influences 24-h Muscle Protein Synthesis in Healthy Adults," *The Journal of Nutrition* 144, 6 (2014): 876–80.

18 M.P. Judge et al., "Maternal Consumption of a DHA-Containing Functional Food Benefits Infant Sleep Patterning: An Early Neurodevelopmental Measure," *Early Human Development* 88, 7 (2012): 531–37.

19 P.C. De Velasco et al., "A Critical Period for Omega-3 Nutritional Supplementation in the Development of the Rodent Visual System," *Brain Research* 1615 (2015): 106–15.

20 M.W. Markhus et al., "Low Omega-3 Index in Pregnancy Is a Possible Biological Risk Factor for Postpartum Depression," *PLOS ONE* 8 (2013): e67617.

21 U. Ramakrishman et al., "Effects of Docosahexaenoic Acid Supplementation during Pregnancy on Gestational Age and Size at Birth: Randomized, Double-Blind, Placebo-Controlled Trial in Mexico," *Food and Nutrition Bulletin* 31, S2 (2010): S108–S116.

22 C. Brandner, "Perinatal Choline Treatment Modifies the Effects of a Visuo-Spatial Attractive Cue upon Spatial Memory in Naive Adult Rats," *Brain Research* 928 (2002): 85–95.

23 S.H. Zeisel et al., "Choline: An Essential Nutrient for Public Health," *Nutrition Reviews* 67, 11 (2009): 615–23.

24 D.D. Alexander et al., "Meta-analysis of Egg Consumption and Risk of Coronary Heart Disease and Stroke," *Journal of the American College of Nutrition* 35, 8 (2016): 704–16.

25 X. Jiang et al., "Maternal Choline Intake Alters the Epigenetic State of Fetal Cortisol-Regulating Genes in Humans," *FASEB Journal* 26, 8 (2012): 3563–74.

26 L. Gallagher, "Nutrition and Pregnancy: Scientists Challenge 'Eat for Two' Myth," Imperial College London, July 28, 2015, http://www3.imperial.ac.uk/newsand-eventspggrp/imperialcollege/newssummary/news_28-7-2015-11-30-23.

Chapter 9: Supplements and Pregnancy

1 B. Worthington-Roberts, "The Role of Nutrition in Pregnancy Course and Outcome," *Journal of Environmental Pathology, Toxicology and Oncology* 5, 6 (1985): 1–80.

2 M.K. Georgieff et al., "Nutrition and the Developing Brain: Nutrient Priorities and Measurement," *American Journal of Clinical Nutrition* 85, 2 (2007): 614S–20S.

3 C.N. Purandare, "Maternal Nutritional Deficiencies and Interventions," *Journal of Obstetrics and Gynaecology of India* 62, 6 (2012): 621–23.

4 S.H. Zeisel, "Choline: Needed for Normal Development of Memory," *Journal of the American College of Nutrition* 19, 5 (2000): 528S–31S.

5 K.S. Moghissi, "Risks and Benefits of Nutritional Supplements during Pregnancy," *Obstetrics and Gynecology* 58, 5S (1981): 68S–78S.

6 F. Parisi et al., "Multiple Micronutrient Needs in Pregnancy in Industrialized Countries," *Annals of Nutrition and Metabolism* 65, 1 (2014): 13–21.

7 J.C. McCann and B.N. Ames, "An Overview of Evidence for a Causal Relation between Iron Deficiency during Development and Deficits in Cognitive or Behavioral Function," *American Journal of Clinical Nutrition* 85 (2007): 931–45.

8 J.R. Hunt et al., "Body Iron Excretion by Healthy Men and Women," *American Journal of Clinical Nutrition* 89, 6 (2009): 1792–98.

9   A.E. Czeizel, "The Primary Prevention of Birth Defects: Multivitamins or Folic Acid?" *International Journal of Medical Sciences* 1 (2004): 50–61.

10   J.L. Mills et al., "Maternal Choline Concentrations during Pregnancy and Choline-Related Genetic Variants as Risk Factors for Neural Tube Defects," *American Journal of Clinical Nutrition* 100 (2014): 1069–74.

11   M. Gadgil et al., "Imbalance of Folic Acid and Vitamin B12 Is Associated with Birth Outcome: An Indian Pregnant Women Study," *European Journal of Clinical Nutrition* 68, 6 (2014): 726–29.

12   G. Goedhart et al., "Maternal Vitamin B-12 and Folate Status during Pregnancy and Excessive Infant Crying," *Early Human Development* 87, 4 (2011): 309–14.

13   L. Masucci and R. Goeree, "Vitamin B12 Intramuscular Injections Versus Oral Supplements: A Budget Impact Analysis," *Ontario Health Technology Assessment Series* 13, 24 (2013): 1–24.

14   U.S. National Institutes of Health, *Vitamin B12: Dietary Supplement Fact Sheet*, February 11, 2016, https://ods.od.nih.gov/factsheets/VitaminB12 -HealthProfessional.

15   T.O. Scholl et al., "Low Zinc Intake during Pregnancy: Its Association with Preterm and Very Preterm Delivery," *American Journal of Epidemiology* 137, 10 (1993): 1115–24.

16   K. Bougma et al., "Iodine and Mental Development of Children 5 Years Old and Under: A Systematic Review and Meta-analysis," *Nutrients* 5, 4 (2013): 1384–416.

17   A. Bener and G.F. Hoffmann, "Nutritional Rickets among Children in a Sun Rich Country," *International Journal of Pediatric Endocrinology* 2010 (2010): 410502.

18   P. Mahon et al., "Low Maternal Vitamin D Status and Fetal Bone Development: Cohort Study," *Journal of Bone and Mineral Research* 25, 1 (2010): 14–19.

19   W. Högler, "Complications of Vitamin D Deficiency from the Foetus to the Infant: One Cause, One Prevention, but Who's [*sic*] Responsibility?" *Best Practice and Research: Clinical Endocrinology and Metabolism* 29, 3 (2015): 385–98.

20   D.W. Eyles et al., "Developmental Vitamin D Deficiency Causes Abnormal Brain Development," *Psychoneuroendocrinology* 34S (2009): S247–57.

21   E. Morales et al., "Circulating 25-hydroxyvitamin D3 in Pregnancy and Infant Neuropsychological Development," *Pediatrics* 130, 4 (2012): e913–20.

22   U.S. Centers for Disease Control and Prevention, "Autism Spectrum Disorder: Data and Statistics," July 11, 2016, http://www.cdc.gov/ncbddd/autism/data .html.

23   T. Wang et al., "Serum Concentration of 25-hydroxyvitamin D in Autism Spectrum Disorder: A Systematic Review and Meta-analysis," *European Child and Adolescent Psychiatry* 25, 4 (2016): 341–50.

24   A. Mithal et al., "Global Vitamin D Status and Determinants of Hypovitaminosis D," *Osteoporosis International* 20, 11 (2009): 1807–20.

25   E. Morales et al., "Vitamin D in Pregnancy and Attention Deficit Hyperactivity Disorder-like Symptoms in Childhood," *Epidemiology* 26, 4 (2015): 458–65.

26   A.A.E. Vinkhuyzen et al. "Gestational vitamin D deficiency and autism spectrum disorder," *British Journal of Psychiatry Open* 3, 2 (2017): 85–90.

27 C. Magnusson et al., "Migration and Autism Spectrum Disorder: Population -Based Study," *British Journal of Psychiatry* 201 (2012): 109–15.

28 J.J. McGrath et al., "Vitamin D3—Implications for Brain Development," *Journal of Steroid Biochemistry and Molecular Biology* 89–90, 1–5 (2004): 557–60.

29 P.J. Goodwin, "Vitamin D in Cancer Patients: Above All, Do No Harm," *Journal of Clinical Oncology* 27, 13 (2009): 2117–19.

30 S.J. Whiting et al., "The Vitamin D Status of Canadians Relative to the 2011 Dietary Reference Intakes: An Examination in Children and Adults with and without Supplement Use," *American Journal of Clinical Nutrition* 94, 1 (2011): 128–35.

31 C.L. Wagner et al., "Health Characteristics and Outcomes of Two Randomized Vitamin D Supplementation Trials during Pregnancy: A Combined Analysis," *Journal of Steroid Biochemistry and Molecular Biology* 136 (2013): 313–20.

32 M. Robinson et al., "Low Maternal Serum Vitamin D during Pregnancy and the Risk for Postpartum Depression Symptoms," *Archives of Women's Mental Health* 17, 3 (2014): 213–19.

33 M.I. McBurney et al., "Suboptimal Serum α-Tocopherol Concentrations Observed among Younger Adults and Those Depending Exclusively upon Food Sources, NHANES 2003-20061-3," *PLOS ONE* 10, 8 (2015): e0135510.

34 M.P. Guerrera et al., "Therapeutic Uses of Magnesium," *American Family Physician* 80, 2 (2009): 157–62.

35 K.S. Lee et al., "Decreased Expression of Collagen and Fibronectin Genes in Striae Distensae Tissue," *Clinical and Experimental Dermatology* 19, 4 (1994): 285–88.

36 J.A. Osaikhuwuomwan et al., "Plasma Vitamin C Levels and Risk of Preterm Prelabour Rupture of Membranes," *Archives of Gynecology and Obstetrics* 284, 3 (2011): 593–97.

37 T.I. Shireman et al., "Docosahexaenoic Acid Supplementation (DHA) and the Return on Investment for Pregnancy Outcomes," *Prostaglandins, Leukotrienes and Essential Fatty Acids* 111 (2016): 8–10.

Chapter 10: Prenatal Planning: A Checklist

1 Health Canada, "Do Canadian Adults Meet Their Nutrient Requirements through Food Intake Alone?" 2012, http://www.hc-sc.gc.ca/fn-an/surveill /nutrition/commun/art-nutr-adult-eng.php#a33 (accessed November 25, 2015).

2 A. Soubry, "Epigenetic Inheritance and Evolution: A Paternal Perspective on Dietary Influences," *Progress in Biophysics and Molecular Biology* 118 (2015): 79–85.

3 N. Maconochie et al., "Risk Factors for First Trimester Miscarriage—Results from a UK-Population-Based Case-Control Study," *BJOG* 114, 2 (2007): 170–86.

4 Y.M. Wei et al., "Risk of Adverse Pregnancy Outcomes Stratified for Pre-pregnancy Body Mass Index," *Journal of Maternal-Fetal and Neonatal Medicine* 1 (2015): 1–5.

5 E.H. Yeung et al., "Parental Obesity and Early Childhood Development," *Pediatrics* 139, 2 (2017), pii: e20161459.

6 C.D. Gardner et al., "Micronutrient Quality of Weight-Loss Diets That Focus on

Macronutrients: Results from the A TO Z Study," *American Journal of Clinical Nutrition* 92, 2 (2010): 304–12.

7   M.S. Linna et al., "Pregnancy, Obstetric, and Perinatal Health Outcomes in Eating Disorders," *American Journal of Obstetrics and Gynecology* 211, 4 (2014): 392.e1–e8.

8   S.V. Dean et al., "Preconception Care: Nutritional Risks and Interventions," *Reproductive Health* 11, S3 (2014): S3.

9   B.A. Haider and Z.A. Bhutta, "Multiple-Micronutrient Supplementation for Women during Pregnancy," *Cochrane Database of Systematic Reviews* 2015, 11 (2015): CD004905.

10 A. Stagnaro-Green et al., "Marginal Iodine Status and High Rate of Subclinical Hypothyroidism in Washington DC Women Planning Conception," *Thyroid* 25, 10 (2015): 1151–54.

11 C. Mora-Esteves and D. Shin, "Nutrient Supplementation: Improving Male Fertility Fourfold," *Seminars in Reproductive Medicine* 31, 4 (2013): 293–300.

12 C. Jacques et al., "Long-Term Effects of Prenatal Omega-3 Fatty Acid Intake on Visual Function in School-Age Children," *Journal of Pediatrics* 158 (2011): 83–90.

13 J.E. Chavarro et al., "Trans Fatty Acid Intake Is Inversely Related to Total Sperm Count in Young Healthy Men," *Human Reproduction* (Oxford) 29, 3 (2014): 429–40.

14 I.P. Tzanetakou et al., "Nutrition during Pregnancy and the Effect of Carbohydrates on the Offspring's Metabolic Profile: In Search of the 'Perfect Maternal Diet,'" *Open Cardiovascular Medicine Journal* 5 (2011): 103–9.

15 U. Nurmatov, G. Devereux and A. Sheikh, "Nutrients and Foods for the Primary Prevention of Asthma and Allergy: Systematic Review and Meta-analysis," *Journal of Allergy and Clinical Immunology* 127, 3 (2011): 724–33.

16 G.K. Beauchamp and J.A. Mennella, "Early Flavor Learning and Its Impact on Later Feeding Behavior," *Journal of Pediatric Gastroenterology and Nutrition* 48, S1 (2009): S25–30.

17 S. Goldberg et al., "Egg Consumption and Carotid Atherosclerosis in the Northern Manhattan Study," *Atherosclerosis* 235, 2 (2014): 273–80.

18 L.B. Andersen et al., "Vitamin D Insufficiency Is Associated with Increased Risk of First-Trimester Miscarriage in the Odense Child Cohort," *American Journal of Clinical Nutrition* 102, 3 (2015): 633–38.

19 R.P. Patrick and B.N. Ames, "Vitamin D Hormone Regulates Serotonin Synthesis, Part 1: Relevance for Autism," *FASEB Journal* 28, 6 (2014): 2398–413.

20 B.W. Hollis et al., "Vitamin D Supplementation during Pregnancy: Double -Blind, Randomized Clinical Trial of Safety and Effectiveness," *Journal of Bone and Mineral Research* 26, 10 (2011): 2341–57.

21 E. Morales et al., "Vitamin D in Pregnancy and Attention Deficit Hyperactivity Disorder-like Symptoms in Childhood," *Epidemiology* 26, 4 (2015): 458–65.

22 For example, see International Osteoporosis Foundation, "Calcium Calculator," http://www.iofbonehealth.org/calcium-calculator (accessed November 27, 2015).

23 R.N. Schlegel et al., "Maternal Hypomagnesemia Causes Placental Abnormalities and Fetal and Postnatal Mortality," *Placenta* 36, 7 (2015): 750–58.

24 R. Elin, "Magnesium Metabolism in Health and Disease," *Disease-a-Month* 34 (1988): 161–219.

25 Q. Dai et al., "Dietary Magnesium, Calcium:Magnesium Ratio and Risk of Reflux Oesophagitis, Barrett's Oesophagus and Oesophageal Adenocarcinoma: A Population-Based Case-Control Study," *British Journal of Nutrition* 115, 2 (2016): 342–50.

26 J.A. Osaikhuwuomwan et al., "Plasma Vitamin C Levels and Risk of Preterm Prelabour Rupture of Membranes," *Archives of Gynecology and Obstetrics* 284, 3 (2011): 593–97.

27 E. Gumpricht and S. Rockway, "Can ω-3 Fatty Acids and Tocotrienol-Rich Vitamin E Reduce Symptoms of Neurodevelopmental Disorders?" *Nutrition* 30, 7–8 (2014): 733–38.

28 E.H. Ruder et al., "Female Dietary Antioxidant Intake and Time to Pregnancy among Couples Treated for Unexplained Infertility," *Fertility and Sterility* 101, 3 (2014): 759–66.

29 T.V. Stephens et al., "Protein Requirements of Healthy Pregnant Women during Early and Late Gestation Are Higher Than Current Recommendations," *Journal of Nutrition* 145, 1 (2015): 73–78.

Chapter 11: The Learning Brain: Diet and Academic Success

1 C.B. Ebbeling et al., "Childhood Obesity: Public-Health Crisis, Common Sense Cure," *Lancet* 360 (2002): 473–82.

2 Childhood Obesity Foundation, "Statistics," updated April 2015, http://child-hoodobesityfoundation.ca/what-is-childhood-obesity/statistics.

3 K.G. Noble et al., "Family Income, Parental Education and Brain Structure in Children and Adolescents," *Nature Neuroscience* 18, 5 (2015): 773–78.

4 B.B. Avants et al., "Relation of Childhood Home Environment to Corticl Thickness in Late Adolescence: Specificity of Experience and Timing," *PLOS ONE* 10, 10 (2015): e0138217.

5 T. Smith-Jackson and J.J. Reel, "Freshmen Women and the 'Freshman 15': Perspectives on Prevalence and Causes of College Weight Gain," *Journal of American College Health* 60, 1 (2012): 14–20.

6 Ibid.

7 A. Boak et al., *The Mental Health and Well-Being of Ontario Students, 1991–2013: Detailed OSDUHS Findings*, CAMH Research Document Series no. 38, https://www.camh.ca/en/research/news_and_publications/ontario-student-drug-use-and-health-survey/Documents/2013%20OSDUHS%20Docs/2013OSDUHS_Detailed_MentalHealthReport.pdf (accessed July 24, 2016).

8 J. Hunt and D. Eisenberg, "Mental Health Problems and Help-Seeking Behavior among College Students," *Journal of Adolescent Health* 46, 1 (2010): 3–10.

9 J.D. Salamone and M. Correa, "The Mysterious Motivational Functions of Mesolimbic Dopamine," *Neuron* 76, 3 (2012): 470–85.

10 H.J. Leidy et al., "Consuming High-Protein Soy Snacks Affects Appetite Control, Satiety, and Diet Quality in Young People and Influences Select Aspects of Mood and Cognition," *Journal of Nutrition* 145, 7 (2015): 1614–22.

11 J.M. Bourre, "Effects of Nutrients (in Food) on the Structure and Function of the Nervous System: Update on Dietary Requirements for Brain, Part 1: Micronutrients," *Journal of Nutrition, Health and Aging* 10, 5 (2006): 377–85.

12 D.O. Kennedy, "B Vitamins and the Brain: Mechanisms, Dose and Efficacy—A Review," *Nutrients* 8, 2 (2016): 68.

13 J.D. Tammam et al., "A Randomised Double-Blind Placebo-Controlled Trial Investigating the Behavioural Effects of Vitamin, Mineral and n-3 Fatty Acid Supplementation in Typically Developing Adolescent Schoolchildren," *British Journal of Nutrition* 115, 2 (2016): 361–73.

14 J. Trebatická and Z. Ďuračková, "Psychiatric Disorders and Polyphenols: Can They Be Helpful in Therapy?" *Oxidative Medicine and Cell Longevity* 2015 (2015): 248529.

15 P.J. Nathan et al., "The Neuropharmacology of L-theanine (N-ethyl-L-glutamine): A Possible Neuroprotective and Cognitive Enhancing Agent," *Journal of Herbal Pharmacotherapy* 6, 2 (2006): 21–30.

16 M.R. Lyon et al., "The Effects of L-Theanine (Suntheanine) on Objective Sleep Quality in Boys with Attention Deficit Hyperactivity Disorder (ADHD): A Randomized, Double-blind, Placebo-controlled Clinical Trial," *Alternative Medicine Review* 16, 4 (2011): 348–54.

17 C.M. Carter et al., "Effects of a Few Food Diet in Attention Deficit Disorder," *Archives of Disease in Childhood* 69, 5 (1993): 564–68.

18 M.D. Kendig, "Cognitive and Behavioural Effects of Sugar Consumption in Rodents: A Review," *Appetite* 80 (2014): 41–54.

19 M. Rumbo et al., "Detection and Characterization of Antibodies Specific to Food Antigens (Gliadin, Ovalbumin and β-lactoglobulin) in Human Serum, Saliva, Colostrum and Milk," *Clinical and Experimental Immunology* 112, 3 (1998): 453–58.

20 J.A. Lieberman and S.H. Sicherer, "Diagnosis of Food Allergy: Epicutaneous Skin Tests, in Vitro Tests, and Oral Food Challenge," *Current Allergy and Asthma Reports* 11, 1 (2011): 58–64.

21 T. Vaa, "ADHD and Relative Risk of Accidents in Road Traffic: A Meta-analysis," *Accident; Analysis and Prevention* 62 (2014): 415–25.

22 K. Unno et al., "Anti-Stress Effect of Theanine on Students during Pharmacy Practice: Positive Correlation among Salivary α-Amylase Activity, Trait Anxiety and Subjective Stress," *Pharmacology, Biochemistry and Behavior* 111 (2013): 128–35.

23 D.A. Drachman, "Memory and Cognitive Function in Man: Does the Cholinergic System Have a Specific Role?" *Neurology* 27, 8 (1977): 783.

24 S.E. Bruce et al., "Improvements in Concentration, Working Memory, and Sustained Attention Following Consumption of a Natural Citicoline-Caffeine Beverage," *International Journal of Food Sciences and Nutrition* 65, 8 (2014): 1003–7.

25 E. McGlade et al., "The Effect of Citicoline Supplementation on Motor Speed and Attention in Adolescent Males," *Journal of Attention Disorders*, July 15, 2015, pii: 1087054715593633.

26 J. Bradshaw, "Students Reaching for ADHD Drugs to Deal with Academic Stress," *Globe and Mail*, October 18, 2013, http://www.theglobeandmail.com /news/national/education/drugs-as-study-aid-a-growing-trend-on-campuses /article14945567.

Chapter 12: Into the Workplace

1 D.O. Kennedy et al., "Multivitamins and Minerals Modulate Whole-Body Energy Metabolism and Cerebral Blood-Flow during Cognitive Task Performance: A Double-Blind, Randomised, Placebo-Controlled Trial," *Nutrition and Metabolism* (London) 13 (2016): 11.

2 T. Knight, "Gorilla Natural History," January 2012, http://web.archive.org /web/20120114083413/http://homepage.mac.com/wildlifeweb/gorillas/info /nh.html (accessed July 30, 2016).

3 Smithsonian's National Zoo and Conservation Biology Institute, "Western Lowland Gorilla," fact sheet, https://nationalzoo.si.edu/animals/western-low land-gorilla.

4 "Gorillas Go Green: Apes Shed Pounds While Doubling Calories on Leafy Diet, Researcher Finds," Science Daily, February 21, 2011, https://www.sciencedaily .com/releases/2011/02/110217091130.htm.

5 S. Savage, "Apes Shed Pounds While Doubling Calories," redOrbit.com, February 17, 2011, http://www.redorbit.com/news/science/1998953/apes_shed _pounds_while_doubling_calories.

6 J.C. Moubarac et al., "Consumption of Ultra-processed Foods Predicts Diet Quality in Canada," *Appetite* 108 (2017): 512–20.

7 S. Lindeberg, "Paleolithic Diets As a Model for Prevention and Treatment of Western Disease," *American Journal of Human Biology* 24, 2 (2012): 110–15.

8 E.M. Steel et al., "Ultra-Processed Foods and Added Sugars in the US Diet: Evidence from a Nationally Representative Cross-Sectional Study," *BMJ Open* 6 (2016): e009892.

9 Standing Senate Committee on Social Affairs, Science and Technology, *Obesity in Canada—A Whole-of-Society Approach for a Healthier Canada*, March 2016, http://www.parl.gc.ca/content/sen/committee/421/SOCI/Reports/2016 -02-25_Revised_report_Obesity_in_Canada_e.pdf.

10 K. Kimura et al., "Theanine Reduces Psychological and Physiological Stress Responses," *Biological Psychology* 74, 1 (2007): 39–45.

11 S.L. Naismith et al., "Circadian Misalignment and Sleep Disruption in Mild Cognitive Impairment," *Journal of Alzheimer's Disease* 38, 4 (2014): 857–66.

12 R.J. Wurtman and J.J. Wurtman, "Brain Serotonin, Carbohydrate-Craving, Obesity and Depression," *Obesity Research* 3, S4 (1995): 477S–80S.

13 J.S. Durmer and D.F. Dinges, "Neurocognitive Consequences of Sleep Deprivation," *Seminars in Neurology* 25, 1 (2005): 117–29.

14   Y. Wei et al., "Synaptic Mechanisms of Memory Consolidation during Sleep Slow Oscillations," *Journal of Neuroscience* 36, 15 (2016): 4231.

15   C.A. Palmer and C.A. Alfano, "Sleep and Emotion Regulation: An Organizing, Integrative Review," *Sleep Medicine Reviews* 2016, pii: S1087-0792(16)00004-6.

16   C.M. Stonnington et al., "Double-Blind Crossover Study of the Cognitive Effects of Lorazepam in Healthy Apolipoprotein E (APOE)-epsilon4 Carriers," *Journal of Clinical Psychiatry* 70, 10 (2009): 1379–84.

17   W. Gomm et al., "Association of Proton Pump Inhibitors with Risk of Dementia: A Pharmacoepidemiological Claims Data Analysis," *JAMA Neurology* 73, 4 (2016): 410–16.

18   T.J. Bunch et al., "Atrial Fibrillation Patients Treated with Long-Term Warfarin Anticoagulation Have Higher Rates of All Dementia Types Compared with Patients Receiving Long-Term Warfarin for Other Indications," *Journal of the American Heart Association* 5, 7 (2016), pii: e003932.

19   S.L. Gray et al., "Cumulative Use of Strong Anticholinergics and Incident Dementia: A Prospective Cohort Study," *JAMA Internal Medicine* 175, 3 (2015): 401–7.

20   A.-C. Granholm et al., "Effects of a Saturated Fat and High Cholesterol Diet on Memory and Hippocampal Morphology in the Middle-Aged Rat," *Journal of Alzheimer's Disease* 14, 2 (2008): 133–45.

21   U.S. Food and Drug Administration, "FDA Drug Safety Communication: Important Safety Label Changes to Cholesterol-Lowering Statin Drugs," February 28, 2012, https://www.fda.gov/Drugs/DrugSafety/ucm293101.htm.

22   A. Macchia et al., "On the Hypothetical Universal Use of Statins in Primary Prevention: An Observational Analysis on Low-Risk Patients and Economic Consequences of a Potential Wide Prescription Rate," *European Journal of Clinical Pharmacology* 71, 4 (2015): 449–59.

Chapter 13: What to Do If Memory Fails

1   Kate Swaffer, "Creating Life with Words: Inspiration, Love and Truth," https://kateswaffer.com.

2   S.N. Young, "Folate and Depression—A Neglected Problem," *Journal of Psychiatry and Neuroscience* 32, 2 (2007): 80–82.

3   R.P. Patrick and B.N. Ames, "Vitamin D and the Omega-3 Fatty Acids Control Serotonin Synthesis and Action, Part 2: Relevance for ADHD, Bipolar Disorder, Schizophrenia, and Impulsive Behavior," *FASEB Journal* 29, 6 (2015): 2207–22.

4   A. Serefko et al., "Magnesium in Depression," *Pharmacological Reports: PR* 65, 3 (2013): 547–54.

5   T.J. Littlejohns et al., "Vitamin D and the Risk of Dementia and Alzheimer Disease," *Neurology* 83, 10 (2014): 920–28.

6   A. Vogiatzoglou et al., "Vitamin B12 Status and Rate of Brain Volume Loss in Community-Dwelling Elderly," *Neurology* 71, 11 (2008): 826–32.

7   E.L. Doets et al., "Interactions between Plasma Concentrations of Folate and Markers of Vitamin B(12) Status with Cognitive Performance in Elderly People

Not Exposed to Folic Acid Fortification: The Hordaland Health Study," *British Journal of Nutrition* 111, 6 (2014): 1085–95.

8   S.H. Zeisel, "Choline: Critical Role During Fetal Development and Dietary Requirements in Adults," *Annual Review of Nutrition* 26 (2006): 229–50.

9   Ibid.

10 M. Fioravanti and A.E. Buckley, "Citicoline (Cognizin) in the Treatment of Cognitive Impairment," *Clinical Interventions in Aging* 1, 3 (2006): 247–51.

11 E. McGlade et al., "Improved Attentional Performance Following Citicoline Administration in Healthy Adult Women," *Food and Nutrition Science* 3, 6 (2012): 769–73.

12 J. Saver and J.L. Kalafut, "Combination Therapies and the Theoretical Limits of Evidence-Based Medicine," *Neuroepidemiology* 20, 2 (2001): 57–64.

13 R.P. Heaney, "Nutrients, Endpoints and the Problem of Proof," *Journal of Nutrition* 138 (2008): 1591–95.

14 Y. Gopalan et al., "Clinical Investigation of the Protective Effects of Palm Vitamin E Tocotrienols on Brain White Matter," *Stroke* 45, 5 (2014): 1422–28.

15 M.W. Dysken et al., "Effect of Vitamin E and Memantine on Functional Decline in Alzheimer Disease: The TEAM-AD VA Cooperative Randomized Trial," *JAMA* 311, 1 (2014): 33–44.

16 T. Morinobu et al., "Measurement of Vitamin E Metabolites by High -Performance Liquid Chromatography during High-Dose Administration of Alpha-tocopherol," *European Journal of Clinical Nutrition* 57, 3 (2003): 410–14.

17 F. Mangialasche et al., "Serum Levels of Vitamin E Forms and Risk of Cognitive Impairment in a Finnish Cohort of Older Adults," *Experimental Gerontology* 48, 12 (2013): 1428.

18 For example, E. Lonn et al., "Effects of Long-Term Vitamin E Supplementation on Cardiovascular Events and Cancer: A Randomized Controlled Trial," *JAMA* 293, 11 (2005): 1338–47.

19 K. Asayama et al., "Double Blind Study of Melatonin Effects on the Sleep-Wake Rhythm, Cognitive and Non-Cognitive Functions in Alzheimer Type Dementia," *Journal of Nippon Medical School* 70, 4 (2003): 334–41.

20 T.C. Bernardo et al., "Physical Exercise and Brain Mitochondrial Fitness: The Possible Role against Alzheimer's Disease," *Brain Pathology* (Zurich) 26, 5 (2016): 648–63.

21 M.C. Morris et al., "MIND Diet Associated with Reduced Incidence of Alzheimer's Disease," *Alzheimer's and Dementia* 11, 9 (2015): 1007–14.

22 F.R. Ellis and S. Nasser, "A Pilot Study of Vitamin B12 in the Treatment of Tiredness," *British Journal of Nutrition* 30 (1973): 277–83.

23 W. Li et al., "Elevation of Brain Magnesium Prevents Synaptic Loss and Reverses Cognitive Deficits in Alzheimer's Disease Mouse Model," *Molecular Brain* 7 (2014): 65.

24 S. Kobayashi and K. Koitabashi, "Effects of Progressive Muscle Relaxation on Cerebral Activity: An fMRI Investigation," *Complementary Therapies in Medicine* 26 (2016): 33–39.

25 D.E. Bredesen, "Reversal of Cognitive Decline: A Novel Therapeutic Program," *Aging* (Albany, NY) 6, 9 (2014): 707–17.

26 M. Wheeler, "Memory Loss Associated with Alzheimer's Reversed for First Time," UCLA Newsroom, October 2, 2014, http://newsroom.ucla.edu/releases/memory-loss-associated-with-alzheimers-reversed-for-first-time.

Chapter 14: Shopping Smarts:
Budget-Conscious Choices at the Grocery Store

1   O. Burger et al., "Human Mortality Improvement in Evolutionary Context," *Proceedings of the National Academy of Sciences of the USA* 109, 44 (2012): 18210–14.

2   E.M. Steele et al., "Ultra-processed Foods and Added Sugars in the US Diet: Evidence from a Nationally Representative Cross-Sectional Study," *BMJ Open* 6 (2016): e009892.

3   J.C. Moubarac et al., "Processed and Ultra-processed Food Products: Consumption Trends in Canada from 1938 to 2011," *Canadian Journal of Dietetic Practice and Research* 75, 1 (2014): 15–21.

4   "Why Processed Food Is Cheaper Than Healthier Options," *Morning Edition*, March 13, 2013, National Public Radio, http://www.npr.org/2013/03/01/173217143/why-process-food-is-cheaper-than-healthier-options.

5   J.C. Moubarac et al., "Consumption of Ultra-Processed Foods Predicts Diet Quality in Canada," *Appetite* 108 (2017): 512–20; E. Martínez Steele et al., "Ultra-Processed Foods and Added Sugars in the U.S. Diet: Evidence from a Nationally Representative Cross-Sectional Study," *BMJ* 6, 3 (2016): e009892.

6   Food Marketing Institute, "Marketing Costs," August 2008, https://www.fmi.org/docs/facts-figures/marketingcosts.pdf.

7   P. Monsivais et al., "Time Spent on Home Food Preparation and Indicators of Healthy Eating," *American Journal of Preventive Medicine* 47, 6 (2014): 796–802.

8   K.L. Haws et al., "Healthy Diets Make Empty Wallets: The Healthy = Expensive Intuition," *Journal of Consumer Research* 43, 6 (2017): 992–1007.

9   C.C. Tangney et al., "Relation of DASH- and Mediterranean-like Dietary Patterns to Cognitive Decline in Older Persons," *Neurology* 83, 16 (2014): 1410–16.

10 M.C. Morris et al., "MIND Diet Associated with Reduced Incidence of Alzheimer's Disease," *Alzheimer's and Dementia* 11, 9 (2015): 1007–14.

11 D. Średnicka-Tober et al., "Higher PUFA and n-3 PUFA, Conjugated Linoleic Acid, α-tocopherol and Iron, but Lower Iodine and Selenium Concentrations in Organic Milk: A Systematic Literature Review and Meta- and Redundancy Analyses," *British Journal of Nutrition* 115 (2016): 1043–60.

12 J.K. Virtanen et al., "Egg Consumption and Risk of Incident Type 2 Diabetes in Men: The Kuopio Ischaemic Heart Disease Risk Factor Study," *American Journal of Clinical Nutrition* 101 (2015): 1088–96.

13 S.C. Larsson et al., "Egg Consumption and Risk of Heart Failure, Myocardial Infarction, and Stroke: Results from 2 Prospective Cohorts," *American Journal of Clinical Nutrition* 102, 5 (2015): 1007–13.

14 T. Ohkuma et al., "Association between Eating Rate and Obesity: A Systematic Review and Meta-analysis," *International Journal of Obesity* (London) 39, 11 (2015): 1589–96.

15 Jonathan Bloom, *American Wasteland: How America Throws Away Nearly Half of Its Food (and What We Can Do about It)* (Cambridge MA: Da Capo Press, 2010).

Chapter 15: Supplement Protocols

1   S. Mayor, "People Taking Proton Pump Inhibitors May Have Increased Risk of Myocardial Infarction, Study Shows," *BMJ* 350 (2015): h3220.

2   J.J. Cannell et al., "Diagnosis and Treatment of Vitamin D Deficiency," *Expert Opinion on Pharmacotherapy* 9, 1 (2008): 107–18.

3   M.J. Bolland et al., "Effect of Calcium Supplements on Risk of Myocardial Infarction and Cardiovascular Events: Meta-analysis," *BMJ* 341 (2010): c3691.

4   J.R. Marier, "Magnesium Content of the Food Supply in the Modern-Day World," *Magnesium* 5, 1 (1986): 1–8.

5   E.J. Brink and A.C. Beynen, "Nutrition and Magnesium Absorption: A Review," *Progress in Food and Nutritional Science* 16, 2 (1992): 125–62.

6   R. Russo and R. Reggiani, "Variability in Antinutritional Compounds in Hempseed Meal of Italian and French Varieties," *Plant* 1, 2 (2013): 25–29.

7   Osteoporosis Canada, "New Vitamin D Guidelines: Physicians Say Canadians Should Be Taking More Supplements," press release, July 14, 2010, http://www.osteoporosis.ca/news/press-releases/new-vitamin-d-guidelines.

8   Health Canada, "Vitamin D and Calcium: Updated Dietary Reference Intakes," March 22, 2012, http://www.hc-sc.gc.ca/fn-an/nutrition/vitamin/vita-d-eng.php.

9   K. Zeratsky, "What Is Vitamin D Toxicity, and Should I Worry about It Since I Take Supplements?" Mayo Clinic, http://www.mayoclinic.org/healthy-lifestyle/nutrition-and-healthy-eating/expert-answers/vitamin-d-toxicity/faq-20058108.

10 T. Judd and G. Kennedy, "Expediency-Based Practice? Medical Students' Reliance on Google and Wikipedia for Biomedical Inquiries," *British Journal of Educational Technology* 42, 2 (2011): 351–60.

11 "Irish Student's Jarre Wiki Hoax Dupes Journalists," Reuters, May 7, 2009, http://www.reuters.com/article/us-wikipedia-hoax-idUSTRE5461ZJ20090507.

12 Harvard T.H. Chan School of Public Health, "Supplement Studies: Sorting Out the Confusion," *Nutrition Source*, https://www.hsph.harvard.edu/nutritionsource/supplement-studies (accessed February 1, 2017).

13 A.R. Martineau et al., "Vitamin D Supplementation to Prevent Acute Respiratory Tract Infections: Systematic Review and Meta-analysis of Individual Participant Data," *BMJ* 356 (2017): i6583.

14 M.J. Bolland and A. Avenell, "Do Vitamin D Supplements Help Prevent Respiratory Tract Infections?" *BMJ* 356 (2017): j456.

15 J.J. Cannell et al., "Epidemic Influenza and Vitamin D," *Epidemiology and Infection* 134, 6 (2006): 1129–40.

16 P.J. Zed et al., "Incidence, Severity and Preventability of Medication-Related Visits to the Emergency Department: A Prospective Study," *CMAJ* 178, 12 (2008): 1563–69.

17 A.C. Ross et al., eds., "Tolerable Upper Intake Levels: Calcium and Vitamin D," chapter 6 in *Dietary Reference Intakes for Calcium and Vitamin D* (Washington, DC: National Academies Press, 2011), https://www.ncbi.nlm.nih.gov/books/NBK56058.

18 Office of Dietary Supplements, National Institutes of Health, "Vitamin K: Fact Sheet for Health Professionals," February 11, 2016, https://ods.od.nih.gov/factsheets/VitaminK-HealthProfessional (accessed March 3, 2017).

19 Micronutrient Information Center, Linus Pauling Institute, Oregon State University, "Vitamin B12," June 4, 2015, http://lpi.oregonstate.edu/mic/vitamins/vitamin-B12 (accessed March 6, 2017).

Index

acetylcholine, 137–38, 178, 189
ADD (attention deficit disorder), 137, 174, 189. *See also* ADHD
Adderall, 179
additives, food, 175–76
ADHD (attention deficit hyperactivity disorder)
   additive-free diet and, 175–76
   in adults, 177–78
   drugs prescribed for, 179
   food allergy testing and, 176
   mercury exposure in pregnancy and, 137
   nutrient deficiency and, 50, 150, 151
   supplements and, 163, 174–75, 177–79, 237–38
adolescents. *See* teenagers and young adults
adrenal glands, 96, 97–98, 99
adrenaline, 20, 48, 62, 99, 102, 105
aging
   chronic degenerative diseases, 77
   cognitive function, 81, 83, 91–92, 206
   high-glycemic foods, 70
   magnesium deficiency, 108
   memory loss, 83, 193–94. *See also* dementia
   need for additional vitamins and minerals, 66, 90, 228
   protein requirements, 72, 135, 224
   tyrosine supplements, 103–104
   vitamin C deficiency, 61
alcohol
   brain health and, 86, 99
   fetal brain development and, 27
   vitamin C and, 61
aldosterone, 98

aggressive behaviour, 53, 60
algal oil, 137, 161
Alhazen, 11
allergies
   childhood, 134, 162
   food, 176–77
   almond(s), 224, 225
   milk, 164, 220
alpha brain waves, 174–75, 188
alpha lipoic acid, 124
alpha-synuclein, 80
alpha-tocopherol, 205, 206
Alzheimer, Alois, 78
Alzheimer's disease. *See also* dementia
   brain cholesterol and, 89
   alcohol and, 86
   development of, 78–79, 84–85, 117
   diabetes and, 80, 85–86
   early-onset, 80
   educational background, 84
   genes and, 84, 88, 90, 193–94
   genetic testing for, 90
   lifespan of patients with, 78
   melatonin and, 207
   mild cognitive impairment and, 81
   prevention of, 40, 208, 218
   risk factors, 42, 49, 60, 70, 88, 93, 123, 189, 202
   vitamin E and, 205
   in women, 79–80
Alzheimer's Research Center (UCLA), 210
Alzheimer's Society, 1
amino acids, 46, 48, 236
amniotic sac, 154, 165

amygdala, 99
anemia, macrocytic, 143
anorexia, 159
antacids, and B12 absorption, 145
antimicrobials, plant-based, 68
antioxidant(s), 48, 67, 123–24, 207
   minerals, 64, 67, 92
   vitamins, 63, 64, 67, 92, 165, 205
anxiety, 28, 52, 95
   and baby's mental health, 132–33
   magnesium gel for, 236
   in post-secondary students, 172–73
   and REM sleep, 191
ApoE (apolipoprotein E) gene, 90, 193–94
apoptosis, 117
apples, 222
Aricept, 202
arterial calcification, 119–20, 232
arthritis, 49, 101–102
artificial colourings and preservatives,
   175–76
ascorbic acid. *See* vitamin C
aspirin, 115
athletic performance, 103
Ativan, 193
Atkins diet, 52
attention deficit disorder. *See* ADD
attention deficit hyperactivity disorder.
   See ADHD
autism spectrum disorder, 35, 149, 151,
   163, 166
avocados, 161, 224
axons, 18, 19, 20, 21, 28

babies. *See* newborns and infants
"baby brain," 162
bananas, 222
Barker, David, 130–31
Baron-Cohen, Simon, 36
beans, 166, 219
beef, 50, 220
benzodiazepine drugs, 193–94
Berger, Hans, 18
berries, 219, 222

beta amyloid, 78
   plaques, 78–79, 84, 90, 93
beta-carotene, 165, 166
biotin, 56
bipolar disorder, 50
birth defects, 141, 143–44
birth weight, 130–32
bisphenol A (BPA), 133
blood-brain barrier (BBB), 21–22
blood clots, 114, 115
blood pressure, 12, 37
   medication, 57
   raised, 80, 108, 116, 122, 146, 208, 218
blood sugar control, 125, 161
blooming (synapse creation), 26–27
blueberries, 126, 219, 222
Blumberg, Jeffrey, 204
body mass index (BMI), 158
bone development, 147–48
bone health, 152, 164, 233
boxing, and brain damage, 112–13
BPA (bisphenol A), 133
brain
   ancients' understanding of, 10–11
   cells, 17, 43, 49–50. *See also* glial cells;
      neurons
   damage. *See* brain trauma
   development, 5, 26–27, 30, 146, 149,
      151, 157, 160, 162, 164
   games, computer-based, 83
   glymphatic system, 87–88
   grey matter (cerebral cortex), 12–13,
      14, 15, 18, 21, 28, 46, 84
   limbic, 98–99
   oxygen and, 43
   reptilian, 98
   rewiring of, 28, 29–30
   scans, 201
   waves, 18–19, 174–75, 188
   white matter, 12, 16, 18, 21, 46, 113, 123, 205
brain mapping, 22–23
The Brain That Changes Itself (Doidge), 28
brain trauma, 16, 28, 112–14, 116
   contact sports and, 112
   nutritional support after, 120, 123–26

bread, 162, 214, 221, 223
breakfast, 222
breastfeeding, 138, 153, 162, 233
Bredesen, Dr. Dale, 210
broccoli, 124, 220–21, 224, 226
bulimia, 159
bullying, 38
burnout, and supplements, 100, 236
busy brain syndrome, 47, 188–89, 210, 236
butter, 219, 220, 224
B vitamins, 90, 91, 144. *See also specific B vitamins*
    activated form, 159
    and brain health, 120
    and mental tasks, 182–83
    in multivitamins, 105, 228
    and physical stamina, 182
    in prenatal multivitamins, 159
    and stress, 104, 173

cafeterias, school and college, 169, 172
caffeine, 42, 99
Cajal, Santiago Ramón y, 17, 18
calcium
    calculators, 164, 233
    channel blockers, 117
    deposits, 119
    and magnesium, 109, 118, 153, 164–65, 233
    supplements, 233
    and vitamin D, 147
    and vitamin K, 119
calories, and nutrient-dense food, 221, 225
Canada
    change of dietary patterns in, 158, 215
    consumption of processed foods in, 216
    food fortification in, 91, 144
    obesity in, 170, 186–87, 216
    vitamin D deficiency in, 147, 151
Canada's Food Guide, 3, 186, 216
cancer, 147, 220, 221, 231
canola oil, 137
Cantu, Dr. Robert, 114
carbohydrates, 58, 70, 125, 134, 221, 223

cardiac arrhythmias, 116
cardiovascular disease. *See* heart disease
Carter, Richard, 148
cauliflower, 138, 220–21, 226
celiac disease, 145, 232
cell theory, 17
cerebellum, 12
cerebral cortex (grey matter), 12–13, 14, 15, 18, 21, 28, 46, 84
cerebrum, 12, 13
cheese, 219, 224
Cheraskin, Dr. Emanuel, 40
chia, 234
A Child of Our Time, 154–55
children. *See also* newborns and infants; teenagers and young adults
    allergies in, 134, 162
    blooming (synapse creation) in, 26–27
    brain injury in, 112, 113–14
    brain size of, 26, 171
    cognitive skills of, 25–26, 27
    empathy development in, 37–39
    fish oil supplements and, 155
    food preferences of, 162
    IQ testing in, 131
    magnesium gel at bedtime, 178
    mental health problems in, 24
    multivitamins for, 243
    school meals for, 169
    semantic memory development in, 171
    trans fats and, 53
    tyrosine supplements and, 236
    vegetable and fruit intake, 125, 222
    vitamin D deficiency in, 147–48, 214, 230
    weight problems in, 158, 170
cholesterol, 51
    HDL, 53, 58–59
    LDL, 53, 58
    medications, 58, 89, 195
    metabolism in brain of, 89
    -rich foods, 139
choline, 137–38, 139
    and memory, 202–203
    supplements, 140, 163

cholinesterase inhibitor drugs, 202, 205
chronic traumatic encephalopathy
(CTE), 113
circadian rhythms, 189, 192
citicoline, 178–79, 203, 208, 238
Cleveland Zoo, 184, 185, 186
clinical trials, randomized (RCTs), 203–204
coconut oil, 53, 126, 161, 185, 224
cod liver oil, 71, 147, 214. *See also* fish oil
supplements
coenzyme Q10 (CoQ10), 48, 101
coffee, 42, 99
cognitive behavioural training, 110
cognitive science, 25, 32
cognitive skills, 25–26, 27, 34
and aging, 81, 83, 91–92, 206
Cognizin, 178, 203
collagen, 61–62, 154, 165
collard greens, 220–21
computer games, brain-training, 83
conceiving, difficulties in, 62, 146, 153,
158, 160, 161, 166
concussion, 114, 178
connective tissue disorders, 62
constipation, 121, 122, 153, 164, 209, 234,
237
contact sports, 112–14
cooking, and healthy diet, 217, 220
copper, 146
"copycat" behaviours, 38
CoQ10 (coenzyme Q10), 48, 101
cortisol, 20, 98–99, 105, 109, 110
cortisone, 98
Cox, Karrissa, 148
cranial nerves, 13, 15
C-reactive protein (CRP), 52, 123
creativity, 22, 102
Crestor, 89
Crick, Sir Francis, 40
Crohn's disease, 145, 232
CRP (C-reactive protein), 52, 123
CT (computerized tomography) scan, 201
CTE (chronic traumatic encephalopathy),
113

dairy products, 50, 145, 164, 233
substitutes for, 164, 233
Dale, Henry, 20
DASH (dietary approaches to stop hypertension), 208, 218
da Vinci, Leonardo, 12
Decade of the Brain, 9–10, 24
dementia, 24, 77
arterial calcification and, 119, 232
B12-deficient, 93, 194
CRP and, 52
drugs for early-stage, 202, 210
frontal lobe, 81, 200–202, 207
mood changes and, 201
nutrition and, 2, 40, 49, 50, 59, 67, 198,
203, 206–207, 208, 210
prevention, 77–78, 90–94, 186, 208
program, 206
risk factors, 2, 46, 80, 85, 88, 95, 194
saturated fat and, 52
semantic memory and, 171, 197
speech problems and, 200, 201
statistics, 1–2
stress and, 95, 207
supplements for, 203, 206, 207
types of, 80–81
vascular, 80
vitamin D deficiency and, 202
dendrites, 17, 18, 28
depression, 24, 95
CRP levels and, 52
vs. dementia, 201
niacin and, 59
nutrition and, 198–99
in post-secondary students, 172, 173
sleep and, 189, 191
supplements and, 199–200
DHA (docosahexaenoic acid), 50, 136, 137,
154, 160, 166, 233
diabetes, gestational, 134, 158, 161
diabetes, type 2, 34
caffeine and, 42
drug treatment for, 145
early warning signs of, 77
eggs and, 221

diabetes (*cont.*)
  hidden hunger and, 170
  low birthweight and, 131
  as risk factor for dementia, 46, 80, 85–86
diet. *See also* nutrition
  Atkins, 52
  crash, 158
  DASH (dietary approaches to stop
    hypertension), 208, 218
  Feingold, 175–76
  high-fat, 53
  low-carbohydrate, 58
  low-fat, low-cholesterol, 51–52, 58, 140,
    161
  Mediterranean, 72, 208, 218
  MIND (Mediterranean-DASH interven-
    tion for neurodegenerative delay),
    70, 208, 218–26
  paleolithic or paleo, 185–86
  of past generations vs. today's, 39
  "veggie-centric," 68, 85, 86–87, 162, 208,
    217, 221–23
  Western-style, 70, 72, 85, 86, 90, 118,
    134, 158, 185, 213
diuretics, 57
dl-alpha-tocopherol, 205, 206, 232
docosahexaenoic acid. *See* DHA
Doidge, Norman, 28
dopamine, 47, 51, 101, 136
  and creativity, 102, 172–73
  and diet, 48–49, 51
  and drug abuse, 172
  maintaining high levels of, 173
  and sleep-wake cycle, 189–90, 191
  and stress, 102–103, 187, 201
  and word recall, 103, 201
drinks, sugar-sweetened, 162
drug abuse, 38, 172
drugs, pharmaceutical, 63. *See also* statin
    drugs
  adverse reactions to, 242
  that increase risk of dementia, 194
  and nutrient depletion, 227

eating disorders, 159
EEG (electroencephalograph), 18–19
  quantitative (qEEG), 22
eggs, 138, 145
  allergy to, 163
  and brain health, 180, 221, 222, 224
  and heart health, 51, 139, 221
  in pregnancy diet, 140, 163
eicosapentaenoic acid. *See* EPA
Einstein, Albert, 21–22
electroencephalograph. *See* EEG
empathy, 34–36
  circuit, 36–37
  development of, 37–38
endorphins, 48, 101
EPA (eicosapentaenoic acid), 50, 136, 137,
    160, 233
epigenetics, 132–33
epilepsy, 19
epinephrine (noradrenaline), 48, 99
Epsom salts, 109
estrogen replacement therapy, 80
eucalyptus oil, 68
eudaimonia, 32
European Food Safety Authority, 243
exercise, 47
  and brain health, 207–208
  excessive, 109
  and nutrient depletion, 150
  for stress management, 109, 199, 200
  and vitamin C, 108
eye development, 160, 165

facial recognition, difficulties with, 92
FAO (Food and Agricultural Organization
    of the United Nations), 61
fast foods, 52, 53, 219
fathers-to-be, 133, 158, 160, 161, 166
fatigue, 60, 96, 98, 103, 153, 235
fats. *See also specific types*
  brain-damaging, 50, 51–52, 219
  brain-healthy, 49–50, 136–39, 161, 224
Feingold, Dr. Ben F., 175
  diet, 175–76

fertility, 62, 146, 153, 158, 160, 161, 166
fertilizers, man-made, 64
fetal brain development, 26, 27, 146
fibre, 134, 162, 184, 185, 186, 221, 227, 234
"fight or flight" hormone, 99
fish, fatty, 49, 71, 72, 219, 224, 225
    and brain development, 145, 160
    and brain health, 50, 85, 91, 136–37, 141
fish oil supplements, 91, 232–33
    alternatives to, 137, 161
    and children, 155, 233
    before pregnancy, 161, 166
    during pregnancy, 136, 160
Fitzgerald, Shane, 240
5-HTP (5-hydroxytryptophan), 192, 193, 237
flaxseed oil, 137
flour, white, 64, 223
Flourens, Marie-Jean-Pierre, 14
folate, 143
folic acid, 56, 91, 142–43, 144
    and B12, 160, 202
    deficiency, and depression, 199
food(s)
    additives, 175–76
    allergy testing, 176–77
    cost of, 216–18
    fortification, 91, 144
    GI ranking of, 45
    high-glycemic, 70, 85, 223
    low-glycemic, 221–22
    nutrient-dense, 221, 225
    organic, 217, 226
    processed, 52–53, 185, 186–87, 190, 215–17, 220, 234
    waste, 225–26
Food and Agricultural Organization of the United Nations (FAO), 61
Food Marketing Institute, 216
football, and brain damage, 112, 113, 114
Framingham Heart Study, 93
free radicals, 43, 48, 63, 67, 92, 222
frontal lobes, 15, 81, 201
frontal lobe dementia, 81, 200–202, 207

fruit
    and brain health, 86–87, 162
    canned, 69
    frozen, 69
    juice, 69, 162, 223
    numbers of servings per day, 68–71, 120, 162, 221–22
    phytochemicals in, 162, 221, 224
    shopping for, 217
    as snack, 222, 224

GABA (gamma-aminobutyric acid), 189
Gage, Phineas, 15–16
Gall, Franz Joseph, 13, 14
gamma-aminobutyric acid (GABA), 189
Gautam, Kul C., 170
genetic makeup. *See also* epigenetics
    and brain health, 33, 34, 88
    tendencies passed down from parents, 122
gestational diabetes, 134, 158, 161
gestational programming, 132
GI. *See* glycemic index
Gilbert, Daniel, 32
Gla proteins, 119
glial cells, 20–21, 22, 87
glucagon, 44
glucose, 30, 44–45, 125, 221
glutathione, 92
glycemic index (GI), 45
    high-glycemic foods, 70, 85, 223
    low-glycemic foods, 221–22
glycogen, 44
glymphatic system, 87–88
goitre, 146
Golgi, Camillo, 18
Gordon, Mary, 38, 39
gorillas, 183, 184–85, 229
grains, 85, 134, 161, 219, 234
GRAS ("generally regarded as safe"), 163, 175
guinea pigs, 106–107
gut microbiome, 5

hallucinations, 81
happiness, 32
    emotional vitality, 33–34
    and genetic makeup, 33
    and mirror neurons, 35
    United Nations study (2011, 2015), 33
hardening of arteries, 119–20, 232
Harlow, Dr. John Martin, 16
HbA1c (hemoglobin), 125
head injury. *See* brain trauma
heartburn, 145, 153, 164, 194
heart disease, 34, 77
    blood cholesterol levels and, 139
    calcium supplements and, 233
    CRP and, 52
    diet and, 49, 51–52, 67, 170, 186, 218, 221, 225
    low birth weight and, 131
    sleep and, 189
hedonia, 32
Heinz Handbook of Nutrition, 4
hemoglobin A1c (HbA1c), 125
hemorrhagic disease, 119
hemp seeds, 234
herbs, 208
hernias, 62
Hibbard, Elizabeth, 143
hidden hunger, 170, 171–72, 174
hippocampus, 26, 83, 99
    development of, 132–33
Hippocrates, 10
histamine, 189
Hooke, Robert, 16–17
hormones, 30, 34
    stress, 48, 96
hospital patients, 62–63
Huntington's disease, 89
hyperactivity. *See* ADHD
hypertension. *See* blood pressure, raised
hypothalamus, 99

Iacoboni, Dr. Marco, 38
immune system, 34, 49, 56, 98, 242, 244
income gap, and brain size, 171

infections, hospital-acquired, 68
inflammation, 49, 50, 53, 63, 98, 117, 123, 222
insomnia, 48, 191, 193, 210, 236–37
Institute of Medicine, 239, 243
insulin, 44–45, 125, 190
    resistance, 45–46, 85
integrative medicine, 110
intelligence, 22, 130, 131–32
intelligence quotient (IQ), 25, 137, 146
    testing, 131
    and vitamin C, 173
Internet, 239–41
intraparietal sulcus, 182
intrinsic factor, 145
iodine, 146, 159–60
iron, 60
    daily requirement, 142

Jarre, Maurice, 240
juvenile delinquency, 38

kale, 220–21
Kaplan, Dr. Bonnie, 65–66
Kennedy, John F., 31
Keys, Ancel, 51
kidneys, 132, 135
Kraft Dinner, 172, 215–16

League of Nations report (1935), 71–72, 214
learning disabilities, 28
lecithin, 163
leftover food, 226
leg(s)
    cramps, 121–22, 153, 164, 165, 178, 193, 234, 236
    restless, 164, 178, 193, 236
lentils, 224, 226
Lewy body disease, 80–81
limbic brain, 98–99
Lipitor, 89
lipoic acid. *See* alpha lipoic acid

liver
  as dietary source of choline, 138
  as dietary source of iron, 214
Loewi, Otto, 20
logical thinking, 22, 27
Losec, 227
low-fat craze, 51, 224
L-theanine, 174–75, 177, 236, 237–38
L-tyrosine, 208, 236, 238
Lukas, Kristen, 184–85
lunch, 222, 226
lycopene, 220
lymphatic system, 87–88

magnesium
  and bowel tolerance, 234–35, 243
  -calcium imbalance, 118, 153, 164–65,
     233
  and constipation, 121, 164, 209, 234
  deficiency, 90, 164, 173, 194
  glycinate, 165, 234
  and head injury, 117–18, 119
  in multivitamins, 228
  and muscle spasms or cramps, 116,
     121, 164, 193, 234
  and sleep, 193
  and stress, 108–109, 118, 200, 234
  and strokes, 116, 117–18, 119, 122
  supplements, 209, 234–35
  topical, 178, 235–36
malnutrition, 61, 170
manganese, 92
margarine, 219
Marmite, 143
Martland, Dr. Harrison, 112
massage therapy, 110
Mayo Clinic, 235, 239
MCI. *See* mild cognitive impairment
meat, 124, 138, 145, 219, 220, 225
media violence, 38
medications. *See* drugs, pharmaceutical
meditation, 188
Mediterranean diet, 72, 208, 218
medulla, 12, 99

melanin, 48, 101
melatonin, 47–48, 123, 192–93, 237
memory
  aging and, 83, 193–94
  cholesterol-lowering drugs and, 89
  choline and, 202–203
  diet and, 68, 138, 218
  improvement of, 207–210, 238
  insufficient B12 and, 91, 202
  long-term, 30, 133
  semantic, 171
  short-term, 30
  stress and, 95, 99, 103, 201
  -targeted supplements, 208
  trans fats and, 53
  working, 30–31, 99
mental retardation, 146
mental tasks, and B vitamins, 182–83
mercury, 137, 160
Metformin, 145
methicillin-resistant Staphylococcus
     aureus (MRSA), 68
methylcobalamin, 160, 209, 229
microbiome, 5
microtubules, 79
mild cognitive impairment (MCI), 81, 91,
     92, 93, 95, 189
milk, 138, 220
Milne, A.A., 177
MIND (Mediterranean-DASH interven-
     tion for neurodegenerative delay),
     70, 208, 218–26
mindful eating, 225
mindfulness-based stress reduction, 110
minerals, 63. *See also specific minerals*
  trace, 63–64, 228
mirror neurons, 35, 37–38
miscarriage, 158, 163
mitochondria, 43, 48, 63
  decay of, 59–60
molybdenum, 228
morning sickness, 135
Moubarac, Dr. Jean-Claude, 186
MRSA (methicillin-resistant
     Staphylococcus aureus), 68

multiple sclerosis, 21, 49, 59
multivitamin and mineral supplements,
    104–105, 123, 165
  children's, 243
  prenatal, 142, 144, 146, 159–60, 164, 165
  selecting, 228–29
mummification, 10–11
muscle
  cramps or spasms, 109, 116, 121
  relaxation technique, 210
musculoskeletal pain, 101–102
myelin, 20–21

nature vs. nurture, 133
necrosis, 116–17
Nedergaard, Dr. Maiken, 88
neuroanatomy, 17
neurogenesis, 26
neuromarketing, 23, 38
neurons, 17–20, 26, 28, 30, 44, 99, 182
  development during pregnancy, 130
  mirror, 35, 37–38
neuroplasticity, 27–28, 30
neurotransmitters, 20, 30, 31, 34, 46, 47,
    62. See also dopamine; serotonin
newborns and infants, 26–27
  birth weight, 130–32
  crying, 144–45
  fine motor skills, 158, 160
  intellectual stimulation of, 171
  mental health of, 132–33
  rickets, 147–48, 214, 230
  sleeping through night, 136, 160
  social skills, 158
  vision of, 160
  and vitamin K, 119
Nexium, 145, 227
niacin (B3), 56, 57–58, 192
  and HDL cholesterol, 58–59
  and mitochondrial decay, 59–60
nicotine, 42. See also smoking
  withdrawal, 190
Niemann-Pick disease, 89
night owls, 189

noradrenaline (epinephrine), 48, 99, 102, 189
norepinephrine. See noradrenaline
nutrients, clinical trials of, 203–204
nutrition. See also diet; specific nutrients
  research, 3, 4, 203–205
  as science, 55
  training of dieticians, 3
  training of medical students, 3, 62, 239
nutritional supplements. See supplements
nuts and seeds, 161, 219, 220, 221, 222, 224
  recommended daily serving, 221

obesity, 80, 85, 133, 134, 140, 186–87, 189
  in children, 158, 170
occipital cortex, 182
oil of oregano, 68
oils, cooking and salad
  canola, 137
  coconut, 53, 126, 161, 185, 224
  flaxseed, 220
  olive, 161, 219, 220, 224
Okinawa, Japan, 91, 225
olfactory bulb, 26
oligodendrocytes, 20–21
olive oil, 161, 219, 220, 224
omega-3, 49–50, 90–91, 93, 173
  and brain development, 53, 136, 137,
    154
  and retinal development, 136
  supplements, 137, 232–33
omega-6, 49, 50
  and brain development, 53, 134, 154
orange juice, 162, 223
organic food, 217, 226
osteoporosis, 62, 120, 164, 232
oxygen, and energy production in brain,
    43–44
Oyebode, Dr. Oyinlola, 69

pain, chronic, 101–102
paleolithic or paleo diet, 185–86
parenting, abusive or unaffectionate, 38
Parkinson's disease, 21, 49, 59, 81, 89, 117, 178

pasta, 162, 214, 221, 223

peanut butter, 166, 220, 224, 225

peanuts, 138

pears, 222

pellagra, 57

penumbra, 115, 116

performance anxiety, 103, 187, 236

personal relationships, importance of, 110

phosphorus, 147

phrenology, 13–14

phytochemicals, 67, 68, 87, 92, 120, 162,
    208, 220, 224

Pick's disease, 81, 82–83

pineal gland, 192

pineapple, 222

plaques, beta amyloid, 78–79, 84, 90, 93

plastics, 133

Pollan, Michael, 215, 216

polyunsaturated fatty acids (PUFAs), 49, 50

Popkin, Barry, 215, 216

postpartum depression, 136, 152

post-traumatic stress disorder (PTSD), 31,
    104–105

potatoes, 162, 214, 221

poultry, 145, 219, 224, 225

PPIs (proton pump inhibitors), 194, 227

prednisone, 98

pre-eclampsia, 158

prefrontal cortex, 30

pregnancy
    anxiety, 132–33, 139–40
    brain fog, 162
    constipation, 153, 237
    and folic acid, 91, 143, 144
    leg cramps, 237
    nutritional deficiencies during, 141,
        145–46, 147–48, 149, 154, 164, 166
    planning for, 133, 157–66
    preterm delivery, 153, 154, 158
    recommended diet before, 130, 133,
        158, 161, 162, 163
    recommended diet during, 130, 132,
        134–35, 136–37, 138–40, 166
    rupture of membranes, premature,
        154, 165

seafood consumption, 137, 160
    stretch marks, 154, 165
    supplements, 142, 144–46, 149, 151–52,
        153, 154, 159–60, 163–65, 237
    vegetarian diet, 161, 166
    weight, 158–59

premenstrual syndrome, 190

presenilin-1 gene, 84

processed foods, 52–53, 185, 186–87, 190,
    215–17, 220, 234

progressive muscle relaxation, 210

prostate cancer, 220

protein, 46–47, 72, 214
    importance during pregnancy, 134–35,
        166
    intake after stroke or TBI, 124
    intake spread throughout day, 135–36,
        224, 225
    shakes, 135

proton pump inhibitors (PPIs), 194, 227

pruning (synapse reduction), 27

psychology, 15

psychopaths, 34–35

PTSD (post-traumatic stress disorder), 31,
    104–105

PUFAs (polyunsaturated fatty acids), 49,
    50, 52

quinine, 121

quinoa, 224, 225

RCTs (randomized clinical trials),
    203–204

reading, and occipital cortex, 182

reflux, 145, 153, 164, 194

relaxation, and brain health, 209–210

reptilian brain, 98

restaurant meals, 223

rice, 162, 214, 221, 223

rickets, 147–48, 214, 230

Ritalin, 179

Roots of Empathy, 38–39

salad dressings, 125, 222, 224
salt, table, 146, 218
saturated fats, 50, 51–52
scans, brain, 201
schizophrenia, 50
scurvy, 60–61, 62
seafood, 139, 145, 224
    mercury contamination in, 137
selenium, 92
Selye, Dr. Hans, 96–97, 110
semantic frontal lobe dementia, 197–98
semantic memory, 171, 197
serotonin, 47–48, 49, 50, 53, 58, 136,
        199
    and sleep-wake cycle, 189–90, 191,
        192
    symptoms of deficiency, 60
serving sizes, 69, 126, 162
sgACC (subgenual anterior cingulate
        cortex), 37
Shaw, George Bernard, 49
shellfish, 137, 145
shopping, food, 217–18
shortness of breath, 153, 164
short-term memory, 30
sleep
    aids, 191–93, 207, 237
    and alcohol, 99
    brain waves during, 19
    and caffeine, 99
    and circadian misalignment, 189
    and darkness of bedroom, 192, 236
    and glymphatic system, 88, 188
    lack of, 48, 188–89, 190–91, 193, 210,
        236–37
    REM (rapid eye movement), 191
    restless, 153
    after stroke or TBI, 123
    -wake cycle, 189–90, 191
sleeping pills, 193, 194
smell, sense of, 26
Smithells, Richard, 143
smoking
    and dementia, 85
    and disease, 42, 85, 133

    and fetal brain development, 27
    giving up, 190
    and vitamin C, 61
smoothies, 125–26, 161, 226
snacks, 173, 190, 221, 222, 224
SOD (superoxide dismutase), 92
soda, 162
soup, 226
soybean oil, 137
spatial intelligence, 138
SPECT (single photon-emission CT)
        scan, 201
spices, 208
spina bifida, 143, 199
spinach, 124, 224
spinal cord injury, 29–30
spine, development of, 143
stage fright, 187
starch, 44, 161–62
statin drugs, 58, 89, 101
    and cloudy thinking, 195
stevia, 162
stir-fries, 226
stress, 97
    B vitamins and, 104, 173
    chronic pain and, 101–102
    effect on brain of, 31, 95, 98–99
    hormones, 62, 96, 97–98, 99, 139
    magnesium and, 108–109, 118, 173
    management, 109–110, 210
    during pregnancy, 132–33, 139–40
    tyrosine supplements for, 102–104,
        187–88, 201, 236
    vitamin supplements for, 65–66, 67,
        104–108
    workplace, 181, 187, 236
Stress without Distress (Selye), 97
stretch marks, 154, 165
stroke, 28, 34, 67
    arterial calcification and, 119, 232
    clot-busting drugs and, 115
    hemorrhagic, 114–15
    ischemic, 114, 116
    low birth weight and, 131
    mini-, 115, 116

stroke (*cont.*)
nutritional support after, 120, 123–26
supplements after, 178, 205, 238
students
diets at exam time, 179–80
post-secondary, 172–74
Stumbling on Happiness (Gilbert), 32
subgenual anterior cingulate cortex
(sgACC), 37
substance abuse, 38, 172
sugar, 44, 45, 125
in fruit juice, 223
in processed foods, 186
suicide, 24, 38, 172
superbugs, 68
"superfoods," 226, 234
superoxide dismutase (SOD), 92
supplements, 2. *See also specific vitamins
and minerals*
buying, 238–39
daily requirements, 66, 227–28
false information about, 239–40
need for healthy people to take, 66–67
regime, 208, 228–36, 244–45
safety of, 242–44
upper limits (UL), 229, 244
surgery, and vitamin C, 108
Swaffer, Kate, 197–98
sweetener, zero-calorie, 162
synapses, 19–20, 26–27, 30
Szent-Györgyi, Albert, 62

Tagamet, 145
tau protein, 78, 79, 81
TBIs (traumatic brain injuries), 28,
112–14, 116
nutritional support after, 120, 123–26
tea, 174–75
tea tree oil, 68
teenagers and young adults
behavioural disorders in, 179
depression and anxiety in, 172–74
drug abuse in, 172
food choices of, 171–72

teeth, 164
temporal lobes, 81
T.H. Chan School of Public Health, 241
theanine. *See* L-theanine
thiamine (B1), 56, 228
thyroid, 146
thyroxine, 48, 101, 146
TIA (transient ischemic attack), 115, 116, 120
tofu, 225
tomatoes, 220
toxins, 133
trans fats, 50, 52–53, 161
transient global amnesia, 195
transient ischemic attack (TIA), 115, 116,
120
traumatic brain injuries. *See* TBIs
tryptophan, 48, 58, 190, 191–92
Tyler-Smith, Chris, 185
tyrosine, 48, 101, 173
supplements, 102–104, 173, 177, 187–
88, 190, 236

ubiquinone (CoQ10), 48, 101
United States, 33, 144, 149
consumption of processed foods in,
216
dietary guidelines, 51
food waste in, 225
obesity in, 170
supplements research, 66–67, 154
upper limits (UL), for essential nutrients,
229, 244
urination, frequent, 153, 164, 193
U.S. Institute of Medicine, 230
U.S. Office of Dietary Supplements, 244

Valium, 193
vancomycin-resistant Enterococcus
(VRE), 68
varicose veins, 165
vascular dementia, 80, 92
vegan diet, 145, 166, 233
vegetarian diet, 137, 145, 161, 166

vegetables
  and brain health, 86–87, 162
  cruciferous, 220–21, 226
  leftover, 226
  number of servings per day, 68–71, 120,
    162, 221–22
  phytochemicals in, 67, 162, 221, 222, 224
  root, 223
  shopping for, 217
  as snack, 222
"veggie-centric" diet, 68, 85, 86–87, 162,
  208, 217, 221–23
Vesalius, Andreas, 12
Victoria, Queen, 13–14
video games, 38
vision, 160
vitamin A, 57, 92
vitamin B1 (thiamine), 56, 228
vitamin B2 (riboflavin), 56
vitamin B3 (niacin/nicotinic acid), 56,
  57–58, 192
  and HDL cholesterol, 58–59
vitamin B5 (pantothenic acid), 56
vitamin B6 (pyridoxine), 56, 105
vitamin B12 (cobalamin), 56, 91–92
  activated form, 160, 228–29
  blood test, 209
  -deficiency dementia, 93, 194
  and folic acid, 160
  food sources of, 145
  injections, 145
  lozenges, 145, 160, 229
  and pregnancy, 144–45, 160
  supplements, 144, 209
  upper limit per day, 244
vitamin C, 57
  and brain health, 62–63, 90, 92, 120
  and collagen production, 61–62, 154,
    165
  and CRP levels, 123
  deficiency, 60–61, 62, 92, 105
  and infertility, 166
  and IQ, 173
  in multivitamins, 228
  and stress, 105–108, 173, 183–84

  supplements, 105, 184, 205, 229
  upper limit per day, 229
vitamin D, 57, 93
  blood test, 209, 231
  as conditionally essential nutrient,
    100–101
  and darker-skinned individuals, 229–30
  deficiency, 71, 93, 147–49, 151, 163, 173,
    202, 229, 230
  and elderly, 229
  and upper respiratory tract infections,
    241–42
  supplements, 152, 164, 209, 230–31
vitamin E, 57, 92, 165–66
  and brain health, 231
  deficiency, 153
  and dementia, 205
  forms of, 205–206
  and infertility, 153, 166
  supplements, 232
vitamin K, 57, 119–20
  and blood clotting, 232
  supplements, 232
  upper limit per day, 244
vitamins. *See also specific vitamins*
  clinical trials of, 203–205
  discovery of, 55–56, 60
  fat-soluble, 57, 232
  water-soluble, 56, 57
  unique needs for, 4, 227–28
vitamin supplements. *See* supplements
VRE (vancomycin-resistant
  Enterococcus), 68

Walker, Dr. Valencia, 149
Ward, Dr. Leanne, 147
warfarin, 194
Warren Anatomical Museum, 15
water pills, 57
weight
  control, 186, 222
  gain, 45, 190, 225
  and lack of sleep, 188–89
  loss, 52

weight (*cont.*)
    -loss surgery, 145
    and pregnancy, 158–59
Wernicke, Carl, 14
wheat bran, 234
whey protein, 124, 126
Wikipedia, 239, 240
Wills, Dr. Lucy, 143
Wilson, E.O., 245
wine, 218
word recall, 103, 201, 238
workplace, 181
    diet at, 182
    performance anxiety at, 187
    stress, 181, 187, 236
    and supplements, 183–84, 189–90
World Health Organization, 1, 85, 233
Wundt, Wilhelm, 15

Yew, Man-Li, 107
yogurt, 222, 224

Zantac, 145
zinc, 92, 145–46, 165, 228